Patterns of Narrative Discourse

A Multicultural, Life Span Approach

Allyssa McCabe

University of Massachusetts Lowell

Lynn S. Bliss

University of Houston

Boston • New York • San Francisco
Mexico City • Montreal • Toronto • London • Madrid • Munich • Paris
Hong Kong • Singapore • Tokyo • Cape Town • Sydney

Executive Editor and Publisher: *Stephen D. Dragin*
Series Editorial Assistant: *Barbara Strickland*
Marketing Manager: *Tara Whorf*
Editorial-Production Administrator: *Beth Houston*
Editorial-Production Service: *Walsh & Associates, Inc.*
Composition and Prepress Buyer: *Linda Cox*
Manufacturing Buyer: *JoAnne Sweeney*
Cover Administrator: *Kristina Mose-Libon*
Electronic Composition: *Publishers' Design and Production Services, Inc.*

For related titles and support materials, visit our online catalog at www.ablongman.com.

Between the time Website information is gathered and then published, it is not unusual for some sites to have closed. Also, the transcription of URLs can result in typographical errors. The publisher would appreciate notification where these errors occur so that they may be corrected in subsequent editions.

Library of Congress Cataloging-in-Publication Data

McCabe, Allyssa.
   Patterns of narrative discourse : a multicultural life span approach / Allyssa McCabe and Lynn S. Bliss.
      p. cm.
   Includes bibliographical references and index.
   ISBN 0-205-33869-0
   1. Discourse analysis, Narrative. 2. Language disorders. I. Bliss, Lynn S.
   II. Title.

P302.7 .M39 2003
401'.41—dc21   2002071727

Printed in the United States of America

10 9 8 7 6 5 4 3 2 1   06 05 04 03 02

For our families.

Contents

Introduction

This book on narrative assessment and intervention is intended for early childhood educators, Head Start professionals, elementary and high school educators, speech-language pathologists, child specialists, adult specialists, individuals in degree programs, and professors of speech-language pathology, special education, developmental psychology, and early childhood education. Our goal is to provide guidelines for assessing narrative, though these guidelines will need to take into account an individual's age and culture, especially. That is to say, readers should not expect this to be a workbook.

Allyssa McCabe is a psychologist who has studied personal narratives for many years, specializing in children's personal narratives from diverse cultures. Lynn Bliss is a professor of speech-language pathology who has conducted research on narratives with Dr. McCabe for the past ten years. Both authors have presented papers on narrative at national meetings. Both authors are from European North American backgrounds and thus have cowritten chapters on individuals of different cultures with full participants of those cultures.

We wish to help prevent two equally problematic mistakes. Specifically, we seek to:

- Prevent misdiagnosis of cultural difference as deficit. What is wrong with misdiagnosing difference as deficit when schools place so much value on a particular European American style of narration? Converting non-European American children to the dominant style of narration may or may not be successful or desirable with fictional stories. Such conversion in the realm of personal narratives is fraught with complications and not a goal to which we personally subscribe. Nor is it clear that professionals should be doing such conversion with otherwise nonimpaired children when so many impaired children need their attention.
- Avoid denying children who need help the help they need. Some individuals may find themselves struggling to communicate at home or in school despite the fact that they have passed tests of vocabulary and syntax. They may have difficulties primarily with discourse that are not addressed by common tests of the other components of language.

The ability to tell a coherent personal narrative is of critical importance in many aspects of a person's life. Children need this ability in order to become accomplished readers and writers. Individuals of all ages and cultural backgrounds need this ability in order to communicate with everyone around them—police officers, doctors, and lawyers as well as family members, neighbors, and friends. The purpose of this book is to train professionals to conduct appropriate and valid narrative assessment so that students and clients will be able to communicate effectively in these contexts. Although all known cultures tell stories, the stories they tell often differ in form from the stories told in other cultures. There are many kinds of good stories.

We will provide readers with the skill to distinguish narrative deficits from cultural variation. While we will focus on the cultural groups about which most information is available (i.e., European North American, African American, Asian American, and Spanish-speaking individuals), we will also present guidelines for dealing with individuals from cultures about which there is not much information available (e.g., Vietnamese, Haitian, and Cambodian). We will offer step-by-step methods for elicitation, scoring, and intervention with personal narratives, the most common type of narrative.

Before we begin our enterprise, we want to highlight a number of important issues, warnings, caveats, and acknowledgments:

- Age must always be taken into account. We expect typical developmental changes in narration, and we will address this broadly by describing what is now known about the development of narrative in various cultures. We will provide examples from preschool children, elementary school children, adolescents, and adults in those cultures.
- When people work with individuals from a culture other than their own, there is no substitute for communication and collaboration with a full participant of that culture (Crago, 1994). We do that in this book and strongly urge readers to do so in their work with students or clients from different cultures. Parents, other professionals, and community leaders are willing to help us do well by their community members, young or old. They understand the need for their help. What is more, educators and clinicians need to examine their own assumptions prior to beginning effective work with individuals from a culture other than their own; that is, counseling individuals from cultures not your own is a complex enterprise (Screen & Anderson, 1994).
- There is much variation among individuals within a culture, let alone different ethnicities broadly grouped together here and elsewhere. We hope readers come away from our book with a questioning sense that cultural issues might have to be taken into account rather than even more prejudgments about what to expect from any given person.
- We have chosen to separate our child samples by ethnicity to enable people unfamiliar with a particular cultural group to become familiar with that culture in some depth.
- We chose to combine our adult samples across ethnic backgrounds for several reasons: We tried to get comparable examples for major acquired disor-

ders, but it did not prove to be possible. We also wanted to balance our prior choice to separate child samples with this inclusive approach.

- We have many samples from individuals with various diagnoses. We caution readers to realize that these samples should not be equated with the diagnosis. There is always heterogeneity among individuals with the same diagnosis.

- As we said, we tried to get comparable examples of major disorders for all cultures, a task that proved to be impossible. We give you what we have to date. We caution readers not to infer that there is any association of disorder with culture, not to infer that some disorders are more common in some cultures.

- This book complements other work we have done. In 1996, the first author published a book called *Chameleon Readers: Teaching Children to Appreciate All Kinds of Good Stories* (McGraw-Hill). That book summarized work up to 1995 in the field as it pertained to the narration of children of various ethnicities. We are happy to say that much more information has become available since that time. The present book picks up where *Chameleon Readers* left off, extending our approach to older individuals and individuals who struggle with various language disorders.

- *The Caveat of Diversity within Groups.* Each of the groups we discuss to some extent identifies itself as a group in the American setting. Labels we use today are inevitably obsolete tomorrow as groups continue to develop distinct cultural identities. The ones we have chosen to use are the ones preferred at this time. The groups we discuss have some storytelling values in common that distinguish them from other groups and so warrant separate consideration. Nonetheless, each of these groups is composed of very different subgroups. While we cannot do sufficient justice to the full scope of human diversity, we will touch on some important within-group differences and commonalities to the extent that these have been documented to date by researchers.

- The most important caveat of all is taken from the Hippocratic oath: First do no harm. We hope to help you avoid mishandling cultural differences between you and your student or client. To ignore such differences or to exaggerate them both have negative consequences. We will show you how to value diversity and include it in clinical contexts.

Acknowledgments

We wish to thank the children, students, and colleagues who have shared their narratives with us.

We would also like to thank the following reviewers for their time and input: Linda M. Bland-Stewart, George Washington University; Yvette D. Hyter, Western Michigan University; and F. Adele Proctor, University of Illinois.

Part 1

Overview

1

Eliciting and Analyzing Personal Narratives

We begin our book on narrative and culture with an oral personal narrative from a 7- year-old Haitian girl (collected, transcribed, and given to the senior author by Yvanne Colinet). She narrated in English because she speaks primarily English. However, she also speaks Creole and a little French, as is typical for Haitian American children. We will call her Michele, though that is not her real name. This narrative is from our personal collection and was offered in the context of a conversation that had included several of our standard prompts but in this case was offered spontaneously.[1]

> (1) Once the crossing guard—you know the crossing guard? (2) (He) lets the stop sign for the bus. (3) The bus has it too. (4) Once he said, "Watch out for the worm!" (5) And there was no worm. (6) Once, you know when it was pouring yesterday, there was so many worms I kept on screaming for real. (6) So, it can get washed off. (7) But I like, "Ewww." (8) There was so many worms. (9) There was a worm in front of me. (10) There was a worm right there (gestures). (11) There was worm right here. (12) There was a hundred worm. (13) And when the kids came out, they said, "I never saw a hundred worm before." (14) It was a lot of worms. (15) When they dig up the ground—I don't know where those worms come from. (16) But the worm don't come from that ground. (17) And it maybe come from somewhere else. (18) It was on floor. (19) It was on the street. (20) It was on the street where, oh my goodness, I was like "Eww,eww,eww,eww,eww,eww!" (21) Once this boy, he said, "There was it was this worm that it was it was it could have—it's not a worm. (22) It evolve into, um yeah. (23) And oh this is pink. (24) This is pink. (25) Pink is my favorite color. (26) And my friend, and he said never saw that once there was so many worms. (27) And there was worms on the street. (28) And there was worm everywhere. (29) There was worms right there, right there, and right there.

---

[1]Here and throughout most of the manuscript we have chosen to display narratives in paragraph form to capture the flow of real discourse rather than to list sentences comprising them.

3

This is a truly hilarious narrative about an experience many of us have had but few have thought to tell about: finding all the worms out, drowned, on the pavement in the springtime. This narrative is a clear account of a specific past experience that is not a typical English-speaking child's narrative (Peterson & McCabe, 1983). No goals, no motivations here, and yet she tells a vibrant narrative in the following ways:

- Vivid description of the worms—how many they were, the fact that they were her favorite color, pink—is provided at the outset and throughout.
- She seeks confirmation that the listener understands about the crossing guard.
- She elaborates her points in such a way that most listeners have to laugh.
- She quotes herself, the crossing guard, other kids, a boy, and her friend, and the use of such reported speech makes a narrative especially vivid.
- She speculates about where all the worms came from and starts to repeat something she has heard about evolution; Michele stops perhaps because she has forgotten the full account of how some "worms" (really caterpillars) "evolve" into butterflies, which is an opportunity for a teacher, parent, or pathologist to provide her with that information again.
- Evaluation pervades the narrative (e.g., "so many worms I kept on screaming for real").
- The repetition and variation of the refrain, "There was worms," is an extremely effective narrative mnemonic device. Several years from now, most listeners/readers will remember the story about all the worms.

We begin with this narrative for a number of reasons. First of all, professionals who look at Michele and hear her speak might jump to the conclusion that the chapter on African American narration in this book would be relevant to understanding whether aspects of her narration are culturally determined. They would be mistaken. Although English is one of her two first languages, Michele's language background and cultural values are Haitian. Her mother was born and raised in Haiti and is Michele's first and most important linguistic influence. She would be an invaluable resource for professionals seeking to work with Michele. What we have to say about African American children whose families have been in the United States for centuries is not relevant to Michele. Thus, the first concern we have is that professionals do not make assumptions about culture. They need to seek information about a person's cultural background to determine whether culture is relevant, and how culture might be relevant for the particular speaker in question.

Definitions

Narrative

Narrative is a type of discourse that usually concerns real or imagined memories of something that happened and therefore is often largely told in the past tense (McCabe, 1991). However, there are also hypothetical, future-tense narratives and others given in the historical present. Sometimes events are broadcast as they occur (e.g., sportscasts). Narratives often contain a chronological sequence of events, but one can also find narratives that contain only a single event or those that skip around in time. Although there are musical, pictorial, and silently dramatic narratives, the narratives that will concern us in this book are a kind of language (McCabe, 1991). Narrative is a level of language expertise that is distinct from syntactic, semantic, and phonological levels. That is, atypically developing children's expertise in narrative does not correlate with measures of syntactic and morphological complexity or size of receptive vocabulary (Hemphill, Uccelli, Winner, & Chang, 2002).

Coherence

Coherence is a judgment we make, formally or informally, about how well put together a piece of discourse is. A narrative is coherent if it is "composed of relevant turns that are thematically related" (Gleason & Ratner, 1998, p. G3). The general judgment of coherence involves several specific dimensions, which we will attempt to specify in the instrument we will present in this book, the narrative assessment profile.

Types of Discourse and Narrative

We will consider this topic in detail in Chapter 7. However, some mention of the variety of discourse needs to be made here. Movie and story retellings, spontaneous fiction in response to story stems, and personal narratives are the major types of narrative that have been explored in research and practice with children and adults. Narrative discourse has received most attention; oral expository or explanatory discourse has received relatively scant attention, though some have considered it (e.g., Beals & Snow, 1994). In fact, this latter type of discourse has received so much less attention than narrative that it is called various names. For example, Bruner (1986) called such logical and scientific description and explanation *paradigmatic* thinking.

In this book, we will focus on the realm of personal narratives because these narratives are relevant to individuals of all ages. They are a means of connecting to other people around us. The extent to which we know another person's important life stories is a pretty good gauge of our intimacy with that person.

Narratives serve many other functions, some of which will be explored in more detail in Chapter 2. Most important among such functions is that narratives enable us to *make sense of our experience*. To understand this better, imagine that you have just had a car accident. The first time somebody asks you what happened, you will be likely to tell a disjointed, somewhat incoherent account of the event. After you have told the story to a number of supportive listeners who have asked questions about the parts you left out, your account will improve in coherence. And you will feel that you really know what happened.

When we tell narratives of personal experience—the genre that we primarily focus on in this book—we also *represent ourselves* in a particular light. That is, we show ourselves to be victims or responsible human beings, jokesters, scoundrels, heros, or a little of all of these. We often alter our representation of ourselves when, for example, telling about an experience to a parent versus a friend.

Narratives are very important in our education as children and adults. Narratives are a memorable way of *making the past present* (O'Brien, 1990) or the abstract concrete. In Chapter 2, we will go into detail about the important role narrative plays in becoming literate. Preschool children are in the process of developing oral narrative skills, a critical prerequisite for literacy. In early elementary school years, personal narrative is a frequent writing assignment ("Write about one important event that happened to you over the summer"), as well as a bridge to stories read in school. Throughout the life span, personal narratives are necessary in communicating with people in the medical profession (e.g., "Tell me how you hurt your knee") and the legal profession ("Tell the court what you witnessed on November 4, 2001), among many other uses, including some on a daily basis. Furthermore, personal narratives, unlike other genres, are integral to all cultures and ages studied to date.

Cultural Composition of Professionals versus Students

According to the 1993 figures compiled by the National Center for Education Statistics (Day, 1996), 86.5 percent of teachers are "white, non-Hispanic," hereafter known as European North American. According to the American Speech-Hearing-Language Association (ASHA) Membership Update 2000, 92.3 percent of speech-language pathologists are European North American; only 7.7 percent of 99,000 pathologists certified by ASHA are members of minority groups. Thus, most professionals bring informal values of narration that are based on European traditions. Furthermore, the extent to which we have been formally educated about well-formed stories, we have been educated almost exclusively in the European tradition. We know Aristotle's definition of a good story as having a clear beginning, middle, and end. Even this mild dictum proves problematic in the face of what we have learned about considerable cultural differences in narrative form.

The European North American background of teachers and speech-language pathologists contrasts to the backgrounds of a large and steadily increasing number of their charges. The Condition of Education 2000 reports that in 1998, 37 percent of public school students in grades 1–12 were considered to be part of a minority group, an increase of 15 percent from 1972. This increase was largely due to the growth in the proportion of students who were Hispanic, which was up 9 percentage points from 1972; Hispanic students account for 15 percent of the public school enrollment. African American students account for 17 percent of public school enrollment. The U.S. Bureau of the Census (1996) reports that by 2030, white non-Hispanics will comprise only 60.5 percent of the total population.

This mismatch means that professionals must gain knowledge about and expertise in dealing with children and adults from cultural backgrounds other than their own. Otherwise, abundant evidence to be reviewed suggests that cultural differences may result in misdiagnosis as deficits, a mistake costly to an already overburdened educational system and potentially disastrous to the individual who is misdiagnosed.

Elicitation of Personal Narrative

As we have suggested, we recommend the genre of personal narrative because it is functional and relevant in many contexts. Before we discuss this genre, we need to describe how we elicit personal narratives.

The first author and Carole Peterson (Peterson & McCabe, 1983) have developed a particular method for collecting personal narratives, which we detail below. Professionals must first understand the way that they themselves affect the form of narrative they hear from their clients.

The Conversational Map Elicitation Procedure (McCabe & Rollins, 1994; Peterson & McCabe, 1983) has been widely used to elicit personal narratives from children with typical and impaired language usage (McCabe & Rollins, 1994; Miranda, McCabe, & Bliss, 1998; Peterson & McCabe, 1983). It has also been used and is applicable for adults. The map operates on the principle that children and adults are much more likely to tell a narrative about their own experiences if examiners share one or more about their own experiences first. The professional tells a brief narrative about an experience and then asks open-ended questions of the person being interviewed. The following steps comprise the Conversational Map Elicitation Procedure.

Story Prompt

In informal interactions spontaneous stories typically generate other spontaneous stories (McCabe & Rollins, 1994). Unfortunately, frequently when professionals say to clients, especially young ones, "Tell me about . . .", they are often met with silence. However, if the professional begins to describe a personal experience, the client may be able to relay a similar personal experience. The similarity of experience gives structure to speakers and assists them in providing a personal experience. The content of the personal experience relayed by the professional (story prompt) is not as important as the fact that one is provided. The goal is to ask individuals to talk about meaningful experiences and have them describe specific events, not typical or routine activities. That is, narratives should be distinguished from scripts. The latter involve descriptions of routine events (e.g., going to a fast-food restaurant).

Children are likely to tell their best narratives in response to requests to talk about injuries (Peterson & McCabe, 1983). Some suggested child narrative elicitation prompts are shown in Box 1.1. Adults talk freely about stolen items, car accidents, hospital stays, and locking themselves out, as we have found in our years of interviewing (see Box 1.2).

Collection of Narrative Samples

Not all people will respond equivalently to any narrative prompt. Individuals have all had different experiences. In order to maximize performance, it is advisable to elicit at least three different narratives from an individual. In this manner, the clinician should be able to tap into the upper range of any individual's narrative performance.

Minimize the Speaker's Self-Consciousness. Attention must be removed from the speaker and the narrative exchange in order to collect useful narratives. A successful technique for children is to have them draw a picture while the narrative is elicited (Peterson & McCabe, 1983). In this way, the children do not feel as though they are being interviewed or judged. Note, however, that some individuals who struggle with producing language may find such tasks too distracting.

A procedure that is more successful with adults is to elicit narrative in an informal manner, not during the formal testing itself. Perhaps the narratives can be elicited before testing in a waiting room or a coffee room. The goal is to make the speaker as comfortable as possible.

Do Not Rush the Speaker.   Personal narratives take time. Speakers need to feel at ease to communicate a story. The professional needs to give them time and listen and show real interest in what they have to say. Specifically, some interviewers are uncomfortable when someone does not immediately respond to their questions. We encourage such people to understand that some individuals—particularly

---

BOX 1.1 • *Suggested Child Narrative Elicitation Prompts*

1. Once I broke my arm. I had to go to the doctor's office. She put it in a cast. Have you ever broken anything? Tell me about it.
2. On my way home last night, I saw a car broken down beside the road. It was all banged up and some windows were broken. Have you ever seen anything like that?
3. Last week, I took my grandmother's cat to the vet because it had a sore on its tail. Did you ever take a pet to the vet? What happened?
4. Two weeks ago, I had to go to the hospital to have some x rays taken. It took a long time. It was scary. Have you ever been to the hospital? Tell me about it.
5. Yesterday I spilled a glass of milk while I was eating dinner. The milk went all over the floor and I had to clean it up. Have you ever spilled anything?
6. Last summer I smelled a pretty flower in the garden. There was a bee on the flower. I didn't see it. It stung me right on the nose. Have you ever been stung?
7. My neighbor had his car stolen last night. He went outside and it was gone. He called the police. Have you ever had something stolen?
8. When I was young, my brother and I got into fights all the time. We would scream and yell at each other. Have you ever fought with someone? Tell me about it.
9. See this bandage? Last night I was peeling potatoes and I cut myself with the knife. Have you ever cut yourself?

Prompts to Avoid
1. Birthday parties: Children often respond by giving a generic script of such events.
2. Trips: Children (and adults) will often give a kind of travel itinerary instead of a narrative about some specific exciting event.
3. Experiences about a loved one who died: Children who are otherwise capable narrators may tell confusing and jumbled sequences and omit evaluative information in such narratives.

BOX 1.2 • *Suggested Adult Narrative Elicitation Prompts*

1. On my way home last night, I saw a car accident. Two cars hit each other. There was glass all over the place. Have you ever been in a car accident? (If no, then: Have you ever seen a car accident?).
2. Two weeks ago, I had to go to the hospital to have an operation. I was there for a week. Have you ever been in the hospital?
3. My neighbor had his car stolen last night. He went outside and it was gone. He called the police. Have you ever had something stolen?
4. I had a dog that ran away. One morning I let him outside and he took off and never came back. Have you ever had a pet that ran away? Tell me about it.
5. Yesterday, I was taking care of my friend's little two-month-old son. I brought him back to my house and parked in the shade and carefully locked the doors to my car. The problem was that he was still inside and so were my keys. I had to call my friend who has a spare set of keys to come home from work and open up the car. Have you ever locked yourself out?
6. I was helping my brother out by taking care of his two pet snakes. But the lid of the container he kept them in was loose. When I got up the first morning, the snakes were gone. I had to tell everyone who came to look out for snakes in my house.

young children and impaired people at all ages—require extra time to formulate their responses. Become comfortable waiting a while for a response. Put the other person at ease.

Use of Relatively Neutral Subprompts.   Neutral subprompts are statements or questions that do not refer to the content of a story but serve to encourage the narrator to continue talking. If an examiner asks specific questions, it will not be possible to determine what the speaker can do on his or her own (Peterson & McCabe, 1983). It is often very difficult to resist asking specific questions when a speaker is having a difficult time in constructing a narrative or gives a very brief one. However, in the evaluation phase, it is critical to withhold specific questions and use more neutral subprompts in order to objectively assess an individual's narrative performance. Some examples of effective and ineffective subprompts are shown in Box 1.3.

Cultural Issues.   This method for collecting narratives has been used successfully by numerous researchers and professionals dealing with children, adolescents, and adults in many English and Spanish-speaking countries, from various Asian backgrounds, from South Africa, and from American Indian, Asian American, and African American ethnicities. It has also been used with individuals from deaf cultures. In fact, so far there is no age nor cultural group with whom this method has failed.

BOX 1.3 • *Subprompts*

Effective, Relatively Neutral Subprompts
1. Repeat the speaker's exact words with rising intonation when they pause:
   Client: Then Dad went home.
   Clinician: Then Dad went home?
2. Say, "Uh-huh."
3. Say, "Tell me more" or "Is that all?"
4. Say, "Then what happened."

Examples of Subprompts to Avoid
1. Where did you go?
2. How did you get there?
3. How did you feel about that?
4. That must have been awful or great or scary, etc.
5. When did you come home?

Analyzing Personal Narratives

In this section we will briefly discuss four different approaches to the analysis of narrative: high point, story grammar, stanza analysis, and narrative assessment profile (NAP), the one we focus on in this book. To give readers a feel for how these analyses contrast with each other, we will use each one to analyze the following narrative:

> *Example of oral narrative—8-year-old Japanese girl*
> *(from the personal collection of Masahiko Minami)*
> *Note that words in parentheses were implied, not actually spoken and that the narrative was originally given in Japanese.*
> (1) When (I was) in kindergarten, (2) (I) got (my) leg caught in a bicycle. (3) (I) got a cut here, here and (4) (I) wore a cast for about a month. (5) (I) took a rest for about a week, and (6) (I) went back again. (7) (I) had a cut here. (8) (I) fell off an iron bar. (9) Yeah, (I) had two mouths.

High-Point Microanalysis

Once professionals have collected narratives, they must look at the overall form and determine whether narrative is an area that is strong or weak relative to other areas of speech/language proficiency for a particular client. One analysis that has been recommended to professionals (Hughes, McGillivray, & Schmidek, 1997; McCabe & Rollins, 1994) is based on the work of Labov (1972) and the related high-point analysis employed by Peterson and McCabe (1983). This relatively fine-grained analysis of constituents will be built into a more holistic assessment (adapted from Peterson & McCabe, 1983; and McCabe & Rollins, 1994) of narrative structure in Chapter 7. In this analysis, the constituents shown in Box 1.4 are tracked in narratives of personal experience. Following the blank form is a high-point microanalysis of the Japanese girl's story. High-point analysis highlights evaluation, and Box 1.5 lists many types of evaluation found previously in children's narratives (Peterson & McCabe, 1983).

BOX 1.4 • *Assessment of Constituents*

Name: _____

Age: _____   Date: _____

Does the client's narrative show presence of the following components? If time permits and for purpose of intervention, it is recommended that specific examples of each of these constituents be documented.

___ 1. Openers (e.g., "I remember one time . . ."): _____

___   Abstracts (e.g., "Did I tell you about when I broke my arm?"): _____

___ 2. Orientation/description

Who: _____
What: _____
When: _____
Where: _____

___ 3. Complicating action (how something happened): _____

___ 4. Climax: _____

___ 5. Resolution (e.g., "We went home after that."): _____

___ 6. Evaluation throughout (why things happened; how narrator felt about them; importance of not coming across as cold to significant others; see Box 1.5): _____

___ 7. Closings

—"That's it/all" and other bailouts (if done repeatedly and prematurely, these may reflect an inability or unwillingness to narrate)

—"So I never ever told another lie." Codas are an elegant means of returning discussion of a past event to the present (Labov, 1972).

(cont.)

BOX 1.4 • *Assessment of Constituents, continued*

Name: _____

Age: _8 years_   Date: _____

Does the client's narrative show presence of the following components? If time permits and for purpose of intervention, it is recommended that specific examples of each of these constituents be documented.

_no_ 1. Openers (e.g., "I remember one time . . ."): _____

_no_   Abstracts (e.g., "Did I tell you about when I broke my arm?"): _____

yes 2. Orientation/description

       Who: _____
       What: ____2 (bicycle)_____
       When: ___1; 4 & 5 partially_____
       Where: ___3, 7_____

yes 3. Complicating action (how something happened): _2, 3, 4, 5, 6, 8_____

_?_ 4. Climax: (This category is n ot directly relevant to Japanese children's narration—Chapter 6.)

_?_ 5. Resolution (e.g., "We went home after that."): _possibly 5_____

yes 6. Evaluation throughout (why things happened; how narrator felt about them) _9_____

_no_ 7. Closings

    —"That's it/all" and other bailouts (if done repeatedly and prematurely, these may reflect an inability or unwillingness to narrate)

    —"So I never ever told another lie." Codas are an elegant means of returning discussion of a past event to the present (Labov, 1972).

Story Grammar Analysis

Another approach to analyzing narratives is known as story grammar or episodic analysis. Hughes, McGillivray, and Schmidek (1997) recommend it for analyzing fictional stories but not personal narratives or scripts. Story grammar examines the extent to which stories are structured around the explicit goals of a protagonist. A good narrative, from this point of view, begins with a setting, continues with an

BOX 1.5 • *Evaluations*

Onomatopoeia ("The car went *bang*!)

Stress ("I caught a BIG fish.")

Elongation ("The water was soooo high in the deep end.")

Exclamation ("I jumped!" said in excited tone of voice)

Repetition ("I screamed and I screamed and I cried and I cried.")

Compulsion words ("I always *have* to take a vitamin.")

Similes and metaphors ("His eyes got as big as tomatoes.")

Gratuitous terms ("I just *put* a bandage on it and went back outside.")

Attention-getters ("I got to tell you the important part.")

Words per se ("That stunk.")

Exaggerations and fantasy ("I was so hungry I could eat a house.")

Negatives ("The doctor didn't give me a shot.")

Intentions, purposes, desires, or hopes ("I wanted to go swimming.")

Hypotheses, guesses, inferences, and predictions ("I guess he wanted to do something else.")

Results of high-point action ("The car got totaled.")

Causal explanations ("I hit him because I hate him.")

Objective judgments ("That was a good thing to do.")

Subjective judgments ("I liked that game.")

Facts per se ("I caught the biggest fish.")

Internal emotional states ("I was sad.")

Tangential information ("Ten dollars is a lot of money when you're a little kid.")

—Adapted from Peterson & McCabe, 1983

initiating event or some explicit problem, a character's internal response and plan, the character's attempt to achieve the goal or solve the problem, and the consequence of that attempt. This approach was based on an analysis of Russian folktales by Vladimir Propp (1968) and is thus explicitly tied to the European tradition of storytelling. Though story grammar has been used in analyzing children's personal narratives (Champion, Seymour, & Camarata, 1995; Peterson & McCabe, 1983), it underrates the narratives of, for example, injuries that go untreated. That is, if a child tells a compelling story about a time she was hurt that meets the definition of being a good narrative from other analytical points of view but that involves no goals or solutions to problems, it will be deemed primitive in story grammar (Peterson & McCabe, 1983).

Another concern with the use of story grammar is that a number of studies have found that children with language impairment can produce all key story grammar constituents when retelling a story (e.g., Graybeal, 1981; Griffith, Ripich, & Dastoli, 1986; Hansen, 1978; McConaughy, 1985; Ripich & Griffith, 1988; Strong & Shaver, 1991; Weaver & Dickinson, 1982). In other words, this analysis does not necessarily register difficulties children have with discourse.

Story grammar is perhaps the best known narrative analysis. However, because it often does not discriminate impaired narration and also because of our interest in non-European background speakers, we will not address it further, except to say that it would characterize the Japanese girl's narrative as comprised of two *primitive* structures, the first at best an *abbreviated episode* with no explicit planning to resolve the problem posed by her injury. The second structure would be termed a *reactive sequence* (see Peterson & McCabe, 1983; Stein & Glenn, 1979). Neither structure reaches the level of the complete episode that would be expected from a girl her age were clinicians unmindful of her cultural background. That is to say, European North American 8-year-olds produced complete episodes or even more complex ones in 76 percent of their narrative structures (Peterson & McCabe, 1983, p. 94). In short, story-grammar analysis may be negatively biased toward narratives that are not produced in the European tradition.

Stanza Analysis

This approach to analyzing narratives involves breaking them into sentences or phrases and grouping these phrases into stanzas. That is, a stanza is a group of sentences related by their joint focus on a subtopic of the larger discourse. There are many variations in the procedure for doing this (see Gee, 1991a, 1991b; Hymes, 1981, 1982; Minami & McCabe, 1991). This method seems to illuminate the structure of narratives from some cultures (e.g., Zuni, Japanese, African American), but not others (e.g., European North American and Mexican American; see McCabe, 1996). Teachers may find it useful in teaching children how to break their writing into paragraphs, but speech language pathologists probably would not. Essentially, it involves displaying a story as if it were a prose poem. Contrast the ordinary transcription of the Japanese girl's narrative (page 10) with the following stanza analysis of it; the first stanza pertains to a first injury, the second to the aftermath of that injury, the third to a second injury:

1. When (I was) in kindergarten
2. (I) got (my) leg caught in a bicycle.
3. (I) got a cut here, here and...

4. (I) wore a cast for about a month.
5. (I) took a rest for about a week, and
6. (I) went back again.

7. (I) had a cut here.
8. (I) fell off an iron bar.
9. Yeah, (I) had two mouths.

Stanza analysis reveals what has been found to be the typical clustering of three phrases per subtopic in Japanese children's personal narratives (Minami & McCabe, 1991), as well as potential parallelism of sentence construction. For example, note the parallelism in all nine sentences above, all of which are statements in which the elliptical *I* serves as subject. Stanza analysis often facilitates cross-cultural understanding (e.g., Minami & McCabe, 1991), the major purpose for which it has been used, by allowing individuals outside a culture to see form and pattern in unfamiliar discourse structures. However, because it does not apply equally well to all cultures, we have chosen a different approach.

Our Approach: Narrative Assessment Profile (NAP)

If a clinician determines that an individual's narration is impaired, then which of the many aspects of narration is the most impaired should be identified for intervention. This triage phase will periodically be repeated throughout therapy/intervention. Note that NAP incorporates aspects of high-point analysis (Labov, 1972; Peterson & McCabe, 1983) via the constituents of informativeness.

The narrative assessment profile (NAP) was developed in order to evaluate discourse coherence. It is comprised of six aspects of discourse coherence that are relevant to the study of the narrative discourse of children and adults (Deese, 1984; Peterson & McCabe, 1983). They are topic maintenance, event sequencing, informativeness, referencing, conjunctive cohesion, and fluency.

The first three dimensions represent general aspects of discourse that involve the macrostructure of narratives. Referencing and conjunctive cohesion reflect more specific discourse functions as they pertain to the relationships between utterances. Fluency is included because it reflects manner of production and is frequently impaired in the discourse of children and adults (Deese, 1984; Peterson & McCabe, 1983).

Description and Scoring of Narrative Assessment Profile Dimensions

Topic Maintenance

This dimension refers to how well all utterances in a narrative relate to a central topic. Utterances may be related to a central theme by expansion, continuation, or contradiction. In contrast, utterances that do not maintain a topic may be irrelevant, tangential, vague, or ambiguous. Descriptions of extraneous routine events (e.g., scripts), associated information such as descriptions of plans, likes, dislikes, capabilities, and possibilities represent deviations in topic maintenance that are often found in specific language impaired (SLI) children (Miranda, McCabe, & Bliss, 1994). Some school-aged children with SLI add extraneous material to the ends of their narratives (Merritt & Liles, 1987; Miranda, McCabe, & Bliss, 1995), launching into a description of a toothbrushing regime in the middle of a narrative about a trip, for example.

Event Sequencing

This dimension involves the presentation of events in chronological or logical order. There generally should be a correspondence between the order of events described by a speaker and the real-life ordering of events unless the narrator indicates to the listener that a violation of ordering will occur. Violation of event sequencing results in *leapfrogging,* characterized by an achronological presentation of events and/or omission of critical events (McCabe & Rollins, 1994; Peterson & McCabe, 1983). These qualities impair discourse coherence because a listener may have difficulty keeping track of events that have been described.

Informativeness

This dimension relates to the sense-making process of discourse coherence; it involves three aspects of the completeness and elaboration of a narrative. The first aspect is that kind of narrative information someone such as a police officer would request: the important facts of some specific experience. In other words, does a narrator present sufficient information for a listener to make sense of a narrative? Omissions of crucial information compromise discourse coherence.

Second, informativeness also comprises embellishment of the sort a teacher would request to make a narrative engaging to listeners. Optional details help make a text coherent. Unelaborated narratives will be barely coherent; the listener will understand the gist of an experience but will be unable to fill in all of the details. As we will see, some cultures value elaboration about participants (see Chapter 5 on Spanish-speaking people), whereas others value action (see Chapter 3 on European North American people).

Finally, a fully informative, coherent narrative contains all basic narrative ingredients: description, action, and evaluation (Labov, 1972). Descriptions consist of attributions of people and objects (e.g., "the red barn"). Actions refer to events (e.g., "He tripped on stage"). Evaluation refers to the subjective significance of an event for a speaker (e.g., "We laughed because we thought it was funny"). Narrative contains many kinds of evaluation (e.g., internal states, exclamations, repetitions and negatives; see Box 1.5; Peterson & McCabe, 1983; McCabe & Rollins, 1994). Evaluation is important because it informs the listener of the speaker's feelings about an event and therefore has interpersonal implications. Without evaluation, a speaker may give the impression of being aloof and unfeeling.

Referencing

This dimension involves the adequate identification of individuals, features, and events (Halliday & Hasan, 1976). Individuals or locations need to be identified before pronouns can be used to refer to them. Inappropriate referencing occurs when pronouns are used without prior identification, when nouns are repeated where pronouns would be expected, or when erroneous pronouns are used (e.g., a feminine pronoun for a man). Referencing contributes to discourse coherence because it enables the listener to identify salient individuals, locations, or events.

Conjunctive Cohesion

This dimension involves words (*and, then, because, so, but*) or phrases that link utterances and events. Conjunctions contribute to coherence because they link concepts and discourse functions. Without conjunctions or with inappropriate ones, the listener may not be able to discern relationships between utterances.

The most commonly analyzed cohesion measures assess semantic links between events (Liles, 1985; Merritt & Liles, 1987; Peterson & McCabe, 1983). Specifically, the following cohesive ties have been studied: **coordination** (e.g., the description of a series of events), **temporal** links (e.g., segments in a time sequence), **causality** (e.g., ties that establish a relationship between cause and effect), **enabling** (e.g., meanings that occur in which one event establishes preconditions for another event), and **disjuncture** (e.g., meanings that involve semantic contrasts between two clauses) (Hood & Bloom, 1979; Peterson & McCabe, 1991).

Another aspect of cohesion involves pragmatic links between utterances (Peterson & McCabe, 1992). Pragmatic aspects of cohesion include a variety of discourse functions (Peterson & McCabe, 1992). The following utterances are examples of pragmatic uses of cohesive devises (Peterson & McCabe, 1992, pp. 452–454):

1. *Beginnings* serve to initiate a narrative. Examiner: "I bet you saw the sun come up in the morning." Child: "*But* I saw the zoo. . . ."

2. *Endings* signal the termination of a narrative. One example involves a child's narrative about a car accident and how many people died. He closed his narrative by saying, ". . . .*So* they dead right now too."

3. *Change of focus* forms signal a departure from an established temporal ordering of events in order to insert additional information, as in the utterance "And then I fell down *but* you know what?"

4. A *chronology violation* signals that a sequential ordering of events will be violated. "We went to Florida *but* first we went to Texas."

Fluency

This final dimension of discourse consists of lexical or phrasal interruptions in utterances. Dysfluencies reduce coherence because they interfere with the understanding of a message. False starts refer to abandoned utterances: "My mom took me to the hospital *and said . . .* uh . . . *the doctor said, we, he, might be . . . we're going to . . .* he *has to do. . . .* can't ride his bike in the street." Internal corrections are retracings of words or phrases with corrections: "We went in the water, *went to the lake,* uh *beach,* by, *up* north . . . We went fishing and . . . we caught, we *found* a snail." Repetitions consist of word or phrasal reiterations that are not used for emphasis: "I swim and kick in the water up north and I *swim and kick.*"

NAP Scoring

All of the questions for each dimension should be asked regardless of whether the answer to each question is positive or negative. A "variable" response can also be given; many individuals are not consistent in their discourse abilities. Research using the NAP has shown such analysis to be reliable (interrater reliability correlation coefficients generally exceed .94) with children (Miranda, McCabe, & Bliss, 1998) as well as adults (Biddle, McCabe, & Bliss, 1996).

Note that the use of *appropriate, inappropriate,* and *variable* judgments (Box 1.6) may appear subjective for several reasons. First of all, such responses are not quantitative. To address this concern, Chapter 11 (p. 161) presents a quantitative form of NAP scoring procedure. However, even when we employ the quantitative approach, we refrain from providing specific numerical guidelines regarding how many orientative statements, for example, are enough to warrant a judgment of "appropriate" or "2." This is a deliberate decision on our part, driven by our knowledge that narrative length varies enormously as a function of context, age, gender, and individual temperament. Specification of numerical standards would be impossible given the extent of such variation. Instead, clinicians must consider a narrative as a whole. Does this little (or lengthy) story contain an adequate amount of evaluation, information, etc.—keeping in mind its overall length and scope?

BOX 1.6 • *Narrative Assessment Profile: Scoring Guidelines*

> **Appropriate.** A behavior is considered to be appropriate when the narrative behavior occurs frequently. Inappropriate behaviors are infrequent enough so as not to reduce discourse coherence.
>
> **Inappropriate.** A behavior is considered to be inappropriate when its frequency reduces discourse coherence.
>
> **Variable.** A behavior is considered to be variable when its frequency occasionally reduces discourse coherence but when the client shows some strengths on a particular dimension.
>
> **Needs further study.** Perhaps further questions are needed; possible cultural variation is involved. This response should be noted when a professional is unsure of whether what children are doing is acceptable in their culture. Professionals should seek information from parents or teachers who are full participants in the child's culture before determining a particular child's own standing.

A clinical format for the NAP is shown in Table 1.1. Once a narrative has been elicited and transcribed, the questions shown can be asked to identify a client's areas of strength and weakness.

TABLE 1.1 *Narrative Assessment Profile with European North American Children and Adults (and adapted to individuals of other cultures)*

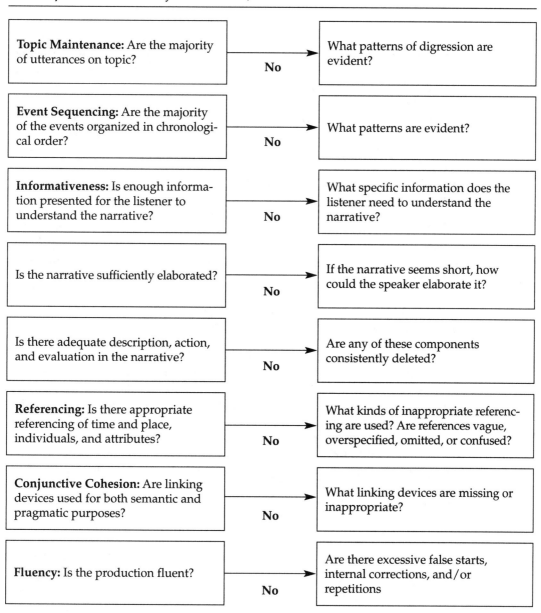

Topic Maintenance: Are the majority of utterances on topic?	No →	What patterns of digression are evident?
Event Sequencing: Are the majority of the events organized in chronological order?	No →	What patterns are evident?
Informativeness: Is enough information presented for the listener to understand the narrative?	No →	What specific information does the listener need to understand the narrative?
Is the narrative sufficiently elaborated?	No →	If the narrative seems short, how could the speaker elaborate it?
Is there adequate description, action, and evaluation in the narrative?	No →	Are any of these components consistently deleted?
Referencing: Is there appropriate referencing of time and place, individuals, and attributes?	No →	What kinds of inappropriate referencing are used? Are references vague, overspecified, omitted, or confused?
Conjunctive Cohesion: Are linking devices used for both semantic and pragmatic purposes?	No →	What linking devices are missing or inappropriate?
Fluency: Is the production fluent?	No →	Are there excessive false starts, internal corrections, and/or repetitions

What follows is an application of the NAP questions to score the Japanese girl's narrative:

Topic Maintenance: As we will explain in Chapter 6, this child maintains topic in the way preferred by Japanese speakers (Minami & McCabe, 1991), which is to combine narration of two or three similar experiences in one narrative.

Event Sequencing: This child sequences two events (2, 3), but again, this dimension is not emphasized in Japanese culture.

Informativeness: As will be discussed in Chapter 6, Japanese listeners are expected to empathize with speakers and to infer relatively more information than many Western listeners, while Japanese speakers are expected to avoid being verbose. We take these cultural values into account in determining that this child is giving enough specific information for us to understand the gist of not one, but two specific experiences.

Is the narrative sufficiently elaborated? The answer is that yes, it is elaborated sufficiently for participants in her culture. Western ears may balk at this, but we ask skeptics to reserve judgment until they read the rest of this book.

Regarding the three types of information, our prior high-point analysis makes clear that the child has given us some description, some action, and some evaluation.

Referencing: This child makes many omissions in referencing, as we have denoted with parentheses in the transcription, and readers may well initially form an impression that she is impaired in this area. However, far from being a sign of pathology, these omissions are a sign that the child is successfully acquiring the values of her culture, summarized in such proverbs as "A talkative person is embarrassing." That is, Japanese speakers often omit pronouns because these can easily be inferred by empathic listeners, and Japanese children are specifically trained to expect that listeners will be empathic, doing far more work in comprehension than Western listeners are accustomed to doing (see Minami & McCabe, 1991, for a review of past research on this issue).

Conjunctive Cohesion: One conjunction appears in the child's narrative; the issues of Japanese cohesion are quite complex, as are translation issues. Suffice it to say that in Japanese, the child's production included appropriate conjunctions (Minami, personal communication).

Fluency: Her production is quite fluent.

In summary, this chapter has defined key terminology and presented details of our preferred method of eliciting personal narratives and the reasons for choosing that genre of narrative. We also contrasted four ways of analyzing a Japanese child's personal narrative.

2

Discourse and Education, Law, and Medicine

In Chapter 1, we reviewed some of the general purposes for narration. In this chapter we will look at the specific uses to which narratives are routinely put. First we will consider this for children, then for adults, though in fact there is no such tidy compartmentalization in the real world.

Narrative and the Acquisition of Literacy

The first kind of evidence that narrative is important to children beginning to acquire reading and writing skills comes from studies that employ some narrative task and relate success in this task to children's literacy skills (Crais & Lorch, 1994; Feagans, 1982; Graesser, Golding, & Long, 1991; Miller, 1990; Snow, 1983; Snow & Dickinson, 1990). To successfully structure narratives is important for a smooth transition to literacy (Heath, 1982, 1983; Michaels, 1991). For example, Paul and Smith (1993) found that narrative skills of 4-year-olds are one of the best predictors of later school outcomes for those children who are at risk for academic and language problems. Feagans and Applebaum (1986) investigated a number of skills in 6- and 7-year-old learning disabled children and found that children demonstrating stronger narrative than syntactic or semantic skills performed better on various standardized academic achievement tests in both reading and math than did peers with weaker narrative skills. Fazio, Naremore, and Connell (1996) investigated low-income children at risk for specific language impairment from kindergarten through second grade. The best kindergarten predictors of those children who were subsequently assigned to remedial education were diminished storytelling and rote memory. Bishop and Edmundson (1987) found that the single best predictor of literacy functioning at age 5½ years was children's performance on a narrative task.

One recent finding comes from the Home-School Study (Tabors, Snow, & Dickinson, 2001). This study followed children enrolled in Head Start from the time they were 3 years old through the seventh grade. These children were representative of the Head Start population in the New England Area and included many African American and Hispanic children as well as European North Americans. This study employed numerous measures of child language and literacy skills over the course of ten years. *Narrative production by these children in kindergarten was one of four measures to correlate significantly with fourth-grade reading comprehension and receptive vocabulary, as well as seventh-grade reading comprehension and receptive vocabulary.*

Given this documentation of a link between narrative ability and subsequent literacy skill, we might ask *why* such a link often surfaces? The answer to that lies in several arenas: (1) The way children tell a story gives listeners, including teachers, an impression about the kind of person they are; (2) the way children habitually tell a story affects their ability to comprehend stories they hear and read; and (3) the way children habitually tell a story is how they will write a story.

Narrative Talk in the Classroom

In considering the many facets of cultural difference in narration, we want to keep in mind two facts: (1) The way people tell a story in one language affects the way they tell a story in another language, and (2) even children draw opinions about what kind of people narrators are based on their discourse style. Children and adults from cultures who value lengthy narratives filled with background information about family members may find the narratives of individuals from cultures who prefer brief narratives to be "cold," while the latter find the narratives of the former to be "rambling." We often misunderstand each other without ever realizing that we do. Recall what we reviewed in Chapter 1 about the increasing mismatch of teachers and students, speech pathologists and clients, and you can see there is increasing potential for misunderstanding around these narrative issues.

The kind of narrative valued in school is one that enables listeners who did not share the experience with the narrator to nonetheless understand what happened. That is, U.S. schools value decontextualized narratives (Bruner, 1986; Cazden, 1985; Snow, 1983). Children who are not able to produce such stand-alone narratives are more apt to be labeled as learning disabled (Roth, 1986).

In view of its importance in predicting the successful acquisition of literacy, *Speaking and Listening for Preschool through Third Grade* (New Standards Project, 2001) has made assessment of oral personal narratives one of its standards for preschool through third-grade children. Where applicable, we will refer to these standards when discussing exemplary narratives. Of additional importance is the fact that "Sharing Events, Telling Stories: Narrative Writing" is one of four aspects of Writing Standard 2 in The New Standards Project on *Reading and Writing, Grade by Grade: Primary Literacy Standards for Kindergarten through Third Grade* (both volumes are available from the National Council for Education and the Economy, *www.ncee.org*). In this very formal way, then, children are expected to meet specific standards for oral personal narration before and then in addition to standards for written narration.

Before we proceed, we need to address the issue of *standards* per se. At the time of writing the present book, educators are more familiar with this term than are speech-language pathologists. In response to this point, we would argue that there is increasing emphasis on the importance of more closely aligning the efforts of pathologists and classroom teachers, and use of a common set of standards should only help to promote this coalition.

Second, many educators are concerned—and rightly so—that standards might well be used to discriminate against children from cultures other than the European North American one. However, the first author of the present volume was directly involved in crafting the narrative standards in the aforementioned volume. Properly crafted and mindful of cultural differences, standards can in fact protect children whose narration may not seem familiar to their European North American teachers but who, once those teachers sit down and look closely, do in fact meet those standards.

Narrative as a Schema for Reading

Much of the material in books read to and by children is narrative of one form or another. One study (Flood, Lapp, & Flood, 1984) examined eight leading basal reading programs to determine the types of writing included in the programs from preprimers to second-grade readers. At all levels examined, the selections were overwhelmingly narrative (56 percent), followed by poetry (25 percent), then exposition (15 percent). Another study (Flood, Lapp, & Nagel, 1991) found that 90 percent of the titles on a list of core works selected for students to read in kindergarten through grade six in twenty-four school districts were fictional (mostly European North American) stories. The stakes for understanding narratives are high: Three of the most common standardized reading tests (i.e., *The Stanford Achievement Test*, *Metropolitan Achievement Test*, and *California Test of Basic Skills*) offer predominantly narrative reading materials (Flood, Lapp, & Flood, 1984).

One of the goals of this book is to sensitize professionals to the fact that some children will bring a sense of story better matched to the stories they encounter at school than other children due in large part to the fact that so many of the narratives at school are European North American in form (Burt & McCabe, 1996). Children from cultures that celebrate different narrative values only rarely get the chance to read narratives that conform to their sense of what makes a good story; that is, serious multicultural literature-based programs are highly unusual in the current education of young children (McCabe, 1996).

Why are cultural differences in narration so important? Children, as well as adults, comprehend and remember more of stories that conform to the structure of the kind of stories they have heard at home (Dube, 1982; Harris, Lee, Hensley & Schoen, 1988; Kintsch & Greene, 1978; Pritchard, 1990). If asked to retell a story from a different culture, individuals of all ages will tend to "misremember" the story to be more like familiar ones. For example, when preschool children heard a story, they retold the story in ways that were distinctive of their cultural background. Specifically, Puerto Rican children recalled far more description and less action than did African American children, who focused more on action than description (John & Berney, 1968).

Consider the findings of a study (Invernizzi & Abouzeid, 1995, pp. 14–16) comparing the story recall of 13- to 14-year-old children from Virginia with children from Ponam Island, Manus Province, Papua, New Guinea. All children were read two Western-style stories: "The Boy Who Cried Wolf" and "Stone Soup." Schooling of Ponam children is in English due to the fact that over 700 different languages exist in Papua, New Guinea. The stories were therefore identical for the two groups, except that cultural tags were adapted for the Ponam children (e.g., "greens" became "kumu"). Invernizzi and Abouzeid found that the Ponam children recalled significantly more than the American children from both stories. However, consider *what* was recalled compared to the original:

Original Version Read to Children in Two Cultures

Once upon a time there was a boy named Kalai who lived on an island with his father and his mother and all his older brothers and sisters. Kalai had no younger brothers or sisters. He was the last born.

As Kalai grew older, he learned to walk, he learned to swim, he learned to help his parents with their work on the island. But he was not happy. Every day he saw his father and his brothers go fishing on the sea, and Kalai wanted to go too. One day as his father and his brothers and sisters got their hooks and lines and glass and spears ready to go fishing, Kalai asked his mother, "Mother, can I go fishing too?"

"No, Kalai," she said, "You are too little. You stay home."

The next day Kalai asked his father, "Father, can I go fishing, too?" His father said, "No Kalai, you are too little to go on the sea. You stay home on the beach."

Kalai was very unhappy, but he stayed home with his mother, and he ate fish and sago every day, and continued to grow bigger.

One day, his mother said to him, "Kalai, you are still too little to go fishing on the sea. But you are big enough to stay home with your grandmother. Today, I am going fishing in the sea with your father and your brothers and your sisters." So Kalai's mother took her glass and spear and got into her canoe and poled away.

Kalai was lonely. He did not know what to do. His grandmother was too old to play games. So he sat down and thought, "How can I make my family come home?" Then he decided. He took a bright red laplap from the clothesline and ran down the beach. He waved the laplap in the air. He ran up and down the beach waving the laplap.

One of Kalai's brothers was fishing, not too far away. He saw the red laplap and came closer. Kalai shouted, "Fire, fire, come home, come home!" Kalai's brother shouted to the others and they all hurried home. When they got home they said to Kalai, "Where is the fire? Hurry! We must put it out quickly."

Kalai said, "There was not any fire. I just wanted you to come home."

Kalai's family was very cross. His father said, "You spoiled my fishing. If you ever tell a lie like that again, I will punish you."

The next day Kalai's father and mother and brothers and sisters went fishing again, and he was left all alone. He was lonely. He was bored. He grabbed the red laplap and ran to the beach, shouting, "Fire, fire!" His family hurried home, but there was no fire.

Now Kalai's family was very, very cross. Kalai was ashamed. He said, "But this time I thought I saw the house on fire. I really thought I did." But Kalai's father knew he had been lying.

The next day Kalai's family went fishing again, and he was alone. He was lonely. He was bored. He lay down and went to sleep under a tree by the side of the cook house. While he slept a little wind came and blew a spark from the fire into the wall of the cook house. Soon the cook house was on fire. Kalai woke and saw the fire. He grabbed his red laplap and ran to the beach. He shouted and shouted. His father saw him and said, "That little liar never learns anything. When I get home I will teach him." Then he went on fishing. Everyone thought Kalai was lying. No one went home.

Now the big house caught fire. Still no one came. The flames grew bigger. Kalai shouted, but no one came. Soon the fire reached the kamal, and that made such a big fire that Kalai's family saw and came home. But it was too late. The cook house, the house, and the kamal were all gone. Kalai cried and cried. He said, "Why did not you come home when I called?" His father said, "Of course we did not come. You lied to us two times before. We did not believe you this time." Kalai's older brother said, "Kalai, do you not know that you must never tell lies? If you tell lies, no one will ever believe you when you tell the truth."

Ponam Retelling (from Invernizzi & Abouzeid, 1995, p. 14)
Once upon a time Kalai and his family they lived on an island. Kalai's mother always carried him everywhere. One day Kalai's mother and father went out fishing. Kalai's mother said, "Kalai you are too small to go out fishing in the sea. You should stay home with your grandfather." Kalai was lonely on the beach. Kalai said, 'How could I get my family home?' He sat down and decided to get his family home. He got his red laplap and ran down to the beach and waved his laplap to his family and said, "Fire, fire." His brother saw his laplap and went home. When they arrived they saw nothing. [END]

American Retelling (from Invernizzi & Abouzeid, 1995, p. 14)
Kalai was running up and down the beach yelling, "Fire, Fire." Everybody came home. The next day the same thing happened. They came home. The next day came but the house caught on fire. He ran up and down the beach but nobody came. Kalai kept waving the flag. Nobody came. Suddenly they saw the flames and the smoke and they came but it was too late. Everything had burnt down to the ground and his brother told him if he kept telling lies that nobody will come when you call for help.

Despite the fact that the American students would be challenged by the notion of what a laplap was, for example, they could infer it to be some article of clothing from the context, and the overall schema of the fable was familiar to them from home and school settings. In other words, American children came to the task prepared to extract what a teacher might have in mind for them to extract because they shared the same sense of story as the author of that version of the story.

The Ponam children, who had been schooled the same amount of time in English stories at school nonetheless have very different narrative values from their

American peers. American children condensed their recalls to the gist of the story (resolution and consequence), while Ponam children elaborated as much as five times the factual details but omitted affect and moral. From a European American point of view, Ponam children wrote detailed factual recalls that seemed to miss the point of both stories. Not one Ponam child included the moral of "The Boy Who Cried Wolf," nor did a Ponam child ever mention the trick that the old man played in "Stone Soup." Ponams do not operate on proverbs, maxims, or anything like that, nor do they see the world as a place full of tricks. These aspects of their culture affect the way they hear stories from other cultures.

Did the Ponam children, then, essentially *misunderstand* the stories? We would argue that they did not. Rather, we would argue that Ponam children *understood* the stories in the way their culture prepared them to understand stories. There are very important implications of this line of research for our purposes:

1. European-based assessments of narrative skill will systematically devalue productions by children from cultures that have different narrative values. Specifically, application of story grammar to the Ponam children's productions made them appear primitive, as Invernizzi and Abouzeid (1995) point out. Care must be taken to avoid bias.
2. Regardless of their cultural background, children with an impaired ability to tell a narrative in turn comprehend and recall less of the stories they hear and read compared to children with more developed narrative skills.
3. The same story will not affect all children equivalently. Many narrative procedures promote the use of stories, prompts, and wordless picture books, as a means of controlling the productions of children. This control is an illusory one due to the fact that children bring different narrative schemas to the reading session.

Narrative as a Schema for Writing

Sarah Michaels (1991) has provided ample documentation of the role that narrative structure—and the mismatch of such structure between teachers and students—plays in children's writing assignments. She examined written compositions over the course of several days and drafts in a sixth-grade classroom. She focused on the compositions that were written over the course of two separate writing assignments, one at the beginning of the school year and one at the end. The data included tape recordings of all whole-group discussions, teacher-student conferences, and nearly all student drafts. She found that at the start of the year most students' first drafts did not meet the teacher's expectations for what makes a good story. In this case the teacher asked the class to write about going to see a circus. In her view, all the compositions should have had a beginning specifying date, place, and the name of the circus to which the class had traveled—information that would make the narrative *decontextualized,* or interpretable to those who had not been on the trip. The teacher then expected a middle section that described and evaluated one particular circus act. Finally, she expected children to conclude with a return to the general—the circus as a whole—with a summary and conclusion.

After a group brainstorming session, a rough first draft, and two writing conferences, one African American girl, with the pseudonym Lewana, produced the following second draft (her spellings have been preserved; example taken from Michaels, 1991, p. 334):

1. On Friday October 19, 1984 all of the six grades went to see Ringling Brothers and Barnum and Bailey Circus at the Bostan garden along with Mr. Strucker and Miss Craig.
2. I thought the antalik Chimps we the cutest animals
3. they had on a white hat, sweater, and pants
4. they were so cute
5. and It was "incredible"
6. because I didn't know that they could walk.
7. They must have had lots of practice and talent
8. because they were good.
9. And I wish I could go again just to see them.
10. **My aunt went Saturday 20, 1984**
11. **and I was mad**
12. **because I couldn't go**
13. **and my sister could.**
14. **I just wanted to go to see the Antalek Chimps**
15. **and when my sister came home**
16. **I asked her what did she like the best**
17. **she said the monkeys.**

Michaels details the numerous interactions and drafts that ensued. However, her most important point concerns the fact that statements 10–17 (in bold print) were rejected by the teacher as belonging to another story. However, to Lewana, whose discourse style will be detailed in Chapter 4, the latter part of her story validated her evaluation of the chimps. That is, the latter half was a most important part of her narrative. The fact that her teacher crossed it out gutted the story from Lewana's point of view. Michaels also noted that by the end of the year all the students' first drafts conformed to the schema the teacher had in mind. Was this a sign of successful education or was it, as Michaels (1991) suggests, instead a "Dismantling of Narrative Structure?"

Do We Outgrow Narrative?

Among educators and speech-language pathologists, not much attention is paid to narratives from adolescents, let alone adults. However, this may well be unfortunate. Consider the case of a classroom in rural Virginia where thirty students aged 14 to 18 years, due to unacceptable behavior, landed. The teacher, Janet McClurg

(Abouzeid & McClurg, under review) found students remarkably engaged when she began a program focusing on taping and transcribing personal narratives. One student commented, "This is the most work I've done in five years," a self-appraisal that was confirmed by his prior teachers (in McCabe, 1996, p. 190).

Adults put personal narrative to numerous important uses. They establish and maintain intimacy with friends and family by exchanging accounts of their experiences, bridging separations by filling others in or reminiscing about evocative shared experiences. Ever since Freud, individuals in psychological distress have sought out therapists to help them make sense of their personal histories so that they can live their lives more fully and with greater peace of mind.

Narrative and Testimony

Although speech-language pathologists and teachers may not find this use immediately relevant to their professional goals, they should be encouraged to realize that, increasingly, even children, including children with special needs, are called upon to offer personal narratives of difficult experiences they have witnessed. That is, one use of personal narrative with very high stakes involves courtroom testimony, and individual and/or cultural limitations in the ability to tell a certain kind of narrative may have profound implications for such children, not to mention adults.

For example, Barry (1991, p. 285) presents numerous examples extracted from real courtroom eyewitness testimony of two very different styles of narrating, one a hyperexplicit style commonly displayed by expert witnesses, such as the member of the homicide squad below. Testimony such as the following is readily accepted by both defense and prosecution lawyers, jury members, and judges:

Q: What did you do upon arriving [at the scene], and about what time did you arrive there?

A: I arrived there approximately—I believe it was 9:45 in the morning—A.M. I was assigned by Sergeant E., who was the officer in charge, to do the scene investigation. It was determined at that time that the state police would be called and I waited until about 12:40—when they arrived and I assisted them in the scene investigation.

Q: Would you tell the jury what you observed about the scene?

A: The scene up in the area—it was in the northeast corner of a fenced-in yard at St. Peter's and in that area was found—located two bodies located near the fence—the northern part of the fence. Also there were several spots of blood, broken two-by-fours or pieces of stick that were located in a circular area where a car had been driven in a kind of figure eight motion.

This witness was more explicit than anyone typically is in everyday life, paying close attention to exact times, directions ("northern part of the fence"), and participants, among other things. Such explicit, believable testimony is distinguished from nonexpert witness testimony (in the same murder trial). In the following excerpt a defense witness who was the girlfriend of the defendant is examined by the defense attorney. She is a friendly witness to the defense attorney, yet even he is unable to keep from interrupting her due to her inexplicit style. Note the lack of detail about objects, the failure to adequately identify the referents of nouns, and the extensive use of pronouns with unclear referents. Note also that elsewhere during her lengthy testimony she was interrupted by the judge and the prosecutor many times (Barry, 1991, pp. 287–288):

A: …which is when E. went out the room and hit him in the head.

Q: Okay, now when E. ran out the room who did he—who did he hit on the head?

…

A: Well both of the men was sittin' on the couch, and he was sayin, "Jest let me go."

Q: Who was sayin' that?

…

A: E. hit him again and then it was two boys—

Q: Who did E. hit? I am not trying—I just want to—

…

Q: When you say T. you are talking about P.S., right"

A: Right.

Q: Maybe you should use P., okay, because that is what has been used throughout this trial.

…

Q: Okay, and what happened then?

A: They just started beating them and at that time E. and …

Q: Okay, when you say "they" can you tell us who was doing the beating and who—first of all, came back in the house?

A: R., E., S., N., T., E., and M.

Q: Okay, and what happened when they got back into the house?

A: Well, they just grabbed him off P. and –

Q: Grabbed who off P.?

A: M.

Q: Okay, grabbed—

A: off P.

Q: Who grabbed M. off P.?

Adults who suffer brain injury that renders them relatively unable to be explicit would find themselves in the same position as this witness, whose testimony was largely discredited because of her inexplicit style of narration.

Narrative and Medicine

There is another common high-stakes use of personal narrative—medicine. Charon (1993) describes the important role of narrative in medical doctor-patient relationships. When doctors ask patients what happened to land them in their office, patients may leave out embarrassing parts of the story. Charon, herself a medical doctor, reports that third-year medical students are taught to describe patients as *reliable* or *unreliable historians*. One medical intern was so irritated at a patient who could not remember details that the doctor felt he needed to know wrote in the hospital chart, "patient ahistoric." This need for stories of a particular kind places adult patients with narrative impairment—who often have considerable need for continued medical treatment—at a great disadvantage as far as the process of receiving optimal treatment is concerned.

In short, personal narrative is important for many reasons to young children and remains important throughout life. Individuals who are compromised in their ability to tell narratives are at great risk for being profoundly misunderstood in the spheres of education, law, and medicine.

Part 2

Typical and Disordered Child Narration in Various Cultures

A. Children with English as a First Language

3

European North American Children

Expected Features of Narration: European North American Children

- Narrative will pertain to a single experience.
- Narrative will contain a fair number of specific actions told in simple past tense and in chronological sequence from the age of 5 years on.
- Narratives often involve some problem or goal that is or is not resolved by the end of the narrative.
- Narratives often begin with some kind of abstract ("Know what? I broke my arm"), provide some orientation as to who, what, when, and where something happened, move into a sequence of actions culminating in a high point or crisis event that is heavily evaluated, mention the resolution of the crisis, and end with a coda that brings narrative past into the present conversation (e.g., "And they dead right now, too").

—Peterson & McCabe, 1983

Example Narratives from Children with Typical Language Development

Children begin to narrate from the age of about 27 months. Their earliest productions consist of one event, usually something that recently happened. A year later, children's best productions are approximately two events long (McCabe & Peterson, 1991).

Preschool-aged children are lengthening their narratives, though at first they tell events in what has been termed a leapfrogging structure (Peterson & McCabe,

1983): that is, the events they tell you are not in sequence, and important information is often left out or seemingly contradictory, as in the following narrative:

> *Preschool oral narrative—4-year-old European North American girl*
> *(from our collection)*
> I got fingers. I got polish on my finger and on my toes. I paint them. I, I did it gooder. My toes. My sister helped me. So my mom didn't, she wanted me to, and I took it off, and, and my, and my mom . . . and and my but then paints my foots and I painted my fingers. My sister did my toes and I and I did my fingernails. And they sharp. When I scratch her, she scratched me back. But I scratch her, and she scratch me back. So I been scratching her. I scratch and she scratched me.

Some key points regarding this narrative are:

- This child produces numerous actions (*paint, did, scratch*), typical of her age, and they are all about one fingernail-painting incident.
- The sequence of actions is confusing, as is also typical of 4-year-old European North Americans (Peterson & McCabe, 1983).
- She includes description ("they sharp") and evaluation ("I did it gooder").
- Referencing is not always clear (e.g., What is the "it" in "I took it off"?).
- There are abundant conjunctions (*and, but, when, so*) usually used for apt semantic reasons; *but* is used either pragmatically to indicate a change of focus in narration or as a mistake. Such usage is typical of children her age.
- Some dysfluencies ("and, and my, and my mom . . . and and my but") are found, but again these are not unusual for a child of her age struggling to produce lengthy discourse.

Consider the following narrative from a 6-year-old European North American boy with typical language development (from our collection):

> Hi Sally. I broke my arm. I was, well, the day [pause] two days ago. I was climbing the tree and I, Well see, I went towards the *low* branch and I, and I got caught with my baving [sic] suit? I dangled my hands down and they got bent because it was like this hard surface under it? Then they bent like in two triangles. But luckily it was my *left* arm that broke.
> [Was everybody home with you?]
> What? *No.* Only my *Mom* was. My mom was in the shower, so I *screamed* for Janie, and Janie goed told my mom.
> [Did you go see Dr. Vincent?]
> I *don't* have Dr. Vincent. I had to go to the hospital and get mm, It was much more worser than you think because I had to get, go into the operation room and I had to get my, And I had to take anesthesia and I had to fall, fall, fall asleep and they bended my arm back and I have my cast on. . . . Do you want to sign my cast?
> [I have to have it on for] six weeks.

Some key points:

- This narrative exemplifies what has been called a "classic" narrative (Peterson & McCabe, 1983), meaning that it begins with an abstract ("I broke my arm"), lays a foundation with orientation as to when the event occurred and ongoing activity at the time ("I was climbing the tree"), and gives a series of events in sequence that culminate in the high point, which is explicitly evaluated ("Then they bent like in two triangles. But luckily it was my *left* arm that broke"). The narrative proceeds to tell us that the incident was resolved by the doctors and ends with a coda, which brings the impact of the incident up to the present time of conversation ("I have my cast on. . . . Do you want to sign my cast?").
- This narrative is appropriate on all six dimensions of the narrative assessment profile (NAP) and exemplifies all the features of narration expected in his culture.
- Note that there are signs that this child is still *developing* typical language: pronunciation differs ("baving" for "bathing"), verbs are overregularized ("bended"), and not all references are accurate ("the tree" should have been "a tree" or "the catalpa tree in the back yard").

In short, problems with narrating events in sequence are considerably reduced by the time children are 5 years old and rarely seen in older children or adults. By the age of 6 years, children tell complete narratives like the preceding one about the broken arm, as well as the one that follows.

> **Elementary school-aged narrative—7½-year-old European North American girl (from our personal collection)**
> I'm, we're lucky we have a big closet. We're lucky we have a shelf way up high. Once Mommy said, "Why'nt you just dust?" And so I got up on that, this doll pan to get polish and a rag. We were polishing and Mommy forgot there was a mouse-trap up there. There wasn't a mouse in it, and guess what? I reached up there and my thumb got caught in it. (*Giggles*) It really scared me. I jumped off the stool. (*Laughs*) Then I went over. Mommy said, "Oh, I'm sorry. I forgot there was one there." (*Giggles*) That did hurt, too.

Some key points about this classic narrative are:

- It begins with orientation as to where and when something happened (in "a closet," at home, "once"), proceeds to build events in sequence ("Mom said . . . I got up . . . We were polishing") to a climax ("my thumb got caught in [the mousetrap]") that is heavily evaluated (by giggling, "It really scared me") and then resolved ("Mommy said, 'Oh, I'm sorry').
- As far as the six dimensions of the NAP are concerned, she does fine. The narrative is centered on one topic, accurately sequenced, and informative. Her references are clear. Conjunctions are used and used appropriately, and the production is fluent.

Adolescent narrative—14-year-, 9-month-old European North American boy (from our collection)

N: We had pitched a tent and had just eaten dinner. Had packed up. I wanted to see the aurora borealis which is the lights in the sky—Northern Lights. And, um, so at around ten. Um, It was before that. It was like eight. I decided I wanted to just go to sleep early so I could wake up at two o'clock and see them—the Northern Lights. So I went into the tent and Dad, and Dad stayed um outside. And uhh I gu. He was just doing stuff outside. He was hiking a little and he came upon a big creature. And then he came back. He said he thought it was a caribou or something before. But then he came into the tent and he saw that there was three bears outside, so he tapped on the outside of the tent and said there was three bears out there, in a kind of whispering voice. I woke up and I was startled. I thought he was joking. I took my camera out and sure enough there about a hundred feet away were two um kind of teenage grizzly bears and a mother. And they were very *well* aware of us. And we kind of waved our hands up above our heads and kind of crouched down a little like they tell you to do in the book.

A: And kind of crashed around a little?

N: Crouched, crouched down a little. Like they tell you to do in the book. And umm, and uh kind of. *One* of them was kind of scared of us and started running away when their mother barked at it. And so he came back and I guess he was trying to prove himself so he crossed the valley which was a little nearer than us. Then he started barking.

A: A little nearer?

N: He crossed the valley really fast and uh, to a place which was nearer to us than he was before. And uh, started going on his hind legs and barking at us and his uh sibling and the mother came by too and they were all kind of barking at us and that was a little scary and then um after about thirty minutes of seeing them they kind of trotted off without touching our food, which was in these little containers—these, uh, bear-resistant containers. And you put them maybe a hundred yards away from your tent and supposedly even if they get to them cause they're on the tundra they can't get into them. And uh, but they didn't even touch them and they just went on their way. And just after that we realized we were on a big batch of blueberries. And that was it.

Some important points about this narrative include:

- This narrative shows that while the basic structure of narrative remains the same as that for the 6- and 7-year-old in the earlier examples, the length has grown substantially. Topic development, event sequencing, and informativeness are far more extensive at this age.
- The narrator takes great care to clarify referents for listeners ("the aurora borealis which is the lights in the sky—Northern Lights"). He monitors himself for references that might be at all unclear ("them—the Northern Lights"). (Note that the unspecified *they* in "like they tell you to do in the book" is a perfectly acceptable colloquial means of referencing experts.)

- Conjunctions are abundant and accurate.
- There are a few typical dysfluencies, which would be true of any speaker with typical language.

Typical Development: Six Dimensions

Topic Maintenance

Topic maintenance emerges in preschool and is mastered during the school-age years. By 2 years, children respond contingently to specific questions and directions (Ervin-Tripp, 1979; Foster, 1986). Topic maintenance abilities improve with increased syntactic abilities (Bloom, Rocissano, & Hood, 1976; Wanska & Bedrosian, 1985). While school-aged children produce semantically congruent utterances (Brinton & Fujiki, 1984), they vary in their ability to maintain a topic throughout the middle childhood years (Brinton & Fujiki, 1984).

Event Sequencing

There generally should be a correspondence between the order of events described by a speaker and the real-life ordering of events unless the narrator indicates to the listener that a violation of ordering will occur. However, at 4 years, children with typical language development often construct leapfrog narratives in which sequence is violated and important information omitted (Peterson & McCabe, 1983). By 5, however, children with TLD are quite capable of sequencing events in their oral narratives (Peterson & McCabe, 1983). From 6 to 9 years, children begin to sequence multiple events within episodes. They are capable of developing well-sequenced chronological summaries of past events, since most European North American cultures value this kind of discourse (Peterson & McCabe, 1983).

Informativeness

Police officer's needs: Do you understand the incident the speaker is trying to relate? The development of informativeness emerges gradually (Peterson & McCabe, 1983). The narratives of children with TLD are characterized by implicitness throughout the primary grades. They tend to omit information that can be easily retrieved by context or topic, such as setting information. From about 4 years of age they are, however, capable of differentiating information that can be omitted from that which listeners cannot infer (Menig-Peterson & McCabe, 1978).

Teacher's goals: Did the speaker give ample detail or just the bare bones of the incident? The extent to which a European North American child elaborates a narrative depends upon many things, especially age and family background. As the examples at the outset of the chapter make clear, as children grow older, they tell lengthier, more elaborate stories. At any age, however, there are considerable differences in the extent to which children elaborate their stories, and these differences stem largely from how much emphasis their parents placed on telling a lengthy story from the time the children were 2 years old (McCabe & Peterson, 1991; see the Appendix for an experimental intervention that also made this point).

Chef's ingredients: Are action, orientation, and evaluation present?   Evaluation is present at 2 years of age—the very beginning of narration—and becomes more frequent in the narratives of older children (Miller & Sperry, 1988; Peterson & McCabe, 1983). Children with TLD from 4 to 9 years of age typically evaluate half of the clauses in their narratives to some degree (Peterson & McCabe, 1983). Narratives of young children also contain action and description (Peterson & McCabe, 1983).

Referencing

The development of referencing varies according to socioeconomic background. Low-income children and adults with TLD frequently use unspecified pronouns (Hemphill, 1989). This usage may reflect a cultural reliance upon the listener to fill in unstated information (Hemphill, 1989). In contrast, middle class speakers value relatively explicit discourse in which the listener is provided with virtually all of the information that is needed to make sense of a narrative (Hemphill, 1989). Referential functions for middle-class children emerge by 3 years (Dasinger & Toupin, 1994). They begin to use pronouns after they have identified people, characteristics, and events (Bamberg, 1987; McGann & Schwartz, 1988). From 5 to 7 years, they are able to indicate changes in references (Bamberg, 1987).

Conjunctive Cohesion

The ability to use a variety of cohesive devices develops throughout the elementary grades (Irwin, 1980). Children use conjunctions (*and, then, because, so, but*) for pragmatic functions (see Chapter 1) as early as they do for semantic ones (Peterson & McCabe, 1991). That is, by 4 years, they are able to use a wide range of conjunctions for both semantic and pragmatic purposes; they rarely violate meanings of conjunctions (Peterson & McCabe, 1991).

Fluency

Fluency is not only a developmental phenomenon; it is influenced by psychosocial factors as well. Increases in dysfluency may be evident with emotionally laden or complex tasks. Fluency is to be expected during early school years. However, dysfluencies tend to increase in the speech of children from 2 to 4 years and decrease in the speech of 5- and 6-year-old children (Ito, 1986). From 6 years to adulthood, there is a continuous decrease in discontinued utterances, repetitions, and fillers (Sabin, Clemmer, O'Connell, & Kaval, 1979).

We turn now to a consideration of the six dimensions with respect to some types of disorders that have been systematically explored.

Group Profile of Children with Specific Language Impairment (SLI)

Topic Maintenance

Some school-aged children with SLI add extraneous material to the ends of their narratives (Merritt & Liles, 1987; Miranda, McCabe, & Bliss, 1998), as if in recognition that they need to say more yet cannot truly extend their commentary on the original topic.

Event Sequencing

Children with SLI have difficulty in marking the temporal ordering of events (Johnston, 1982; Liles, 1985a; Olley, 1989). They may not have mastered temporal terms or concepts (Lucas, 1980) or may not be able to use them to signal the order of events in narratives. Long past the age of 4, children with SLI continue to produce disjointed leapfrog narratives in which events are not presented sequentially and important ones are omitted. In addition, such children may repeat events as a strategy to avoid sequencing additional actions. Retelling is easier than constructing narrative from scratch.

Informativeness

Children with SLI tend to leave out information that pertains to individuals, plans, actions, internal states, and orientation (Liles, 1987; Merritt & Liles, 1987; Sleight & Prinz, 1985, Roth & Spekman, 1986). The listener must fill in missing information (Miranda, McCabe, & Bliss, 1998; Roth & Spekman, 1986). Their narratives may also lack elaboration. While the text can be understood, the absence of optional information makes it difficult for a listener to fully understand the story. Narratives of children with SLI may also contain inaccurate, confusing information. The reason for a failure to be explicit may be a limited awareness of the communication needs of the listener.

Referencing

Children with SLI frequently have different or inadequate referencing abilities (Liles, 1985a, 1985b; Liles, 1987; Olley, 1989). They use fewer personal pronouns and more demonstratives (e.g., *this* and *that*) and nouns to identify individuals than their age-matched peers with TLD (Liles, 1985b). Such differences in referencing may result from delayed development of pronouns in general or a limited ability to maintain reference using pronouns in narrative discourse (Liles, 1985a).

Conjunctive Cohesion

Children with SLI have difficulty in semantically using conjunctions for cohesion (Liles, 1987). They also have a higher incidence of inaccurate ties (Liles, 1985a; 1987). The frequency of inaccurate conjunctions is particularly evident when they attempt to formulate a series of utterances (Purcell & Liles, 1992; Liles, 1987). The origins of this deficit may include lack of comprehension of logical relationships between events, reduced ability to organize information, and inadequate ability to construct oral texts (Liles, 1987).

However, conjunctions that appear to represent semantic errors instead may be used appropriately for pragmatic purposes. For example, a conjunction might be considered to be inappropriate when it begins an utterance without a semantic link to a previous utterance. However, the speaker in fact may be signaling a beginning of a discourse, which would represent a pragmatic discourse function. In the following example, a semantic violation of conjunction usage is evident from an 8-year-old child with SLI: "I just broke my leg and I just fall down on my bike *because* I got hurt." The child has reversed cause and effect meanings. Children with TLD rarely reverse cause and effect in spontaneous conversation (McCabe & Peterson, 1985; Peterson & McCabe, 1992), but this child with SLI did; his use of the conjunction was a pragmatic acknowledgment of this reversal. In the following utterance, from an 8-year-old boy with SLI, the conjunction *but* is used to serve two different functions:

> **Interviewer:**   "Did you ever take an animal to the vet?"
>
> **Child:**   "My little dog and my big dog and my cat *but* my cat been scared *but* he got a shot by its butt 'cause he been mean."

In the first occurrence, *but* is used pragmatically to signal a change of focus. In the second occurrence, *but* reflects a semantic error in which an adversative meaning is indicated instead of the appropriate causal one. In other words, children with SLI might well make fewer errors in conjunctive usage than prior research suggests because no one to date has systematically accounted for their pragmatic usage.

Fluency

Some children with SLI exhibit dysfluencies in their discourse (German & Simon, 1991; MacLachlan & Chapman, 1988). Their dysfluencies are more evident in narration than in nonnarrative discourse (MacLachlan & Chapman, 1988). The incidence of dysfluencies may be related to word-finding deficits (German & Simon, 1991) or to a reduced ability to plan, monitor, and repair utterances (Peterson & McCabe, 1983). Children with SLI appear to monitor meaning relations more than grammatical form (Purcell & Liles, 1992).

Consider the following example of a narrative from a child with SLI, followed by a NAP of that narrative:

Example from 9-year-, 3-month-old European North American, middle-class boy with SLI (from Bliss, McCabe, & Miranda, 1998)

E: Two weeks ago I had to go to the hospital to have some x rays taken. Have you ever been to the hospital?

R: (1) Yeah, I had a x ray because they they're checking on my leg and I was scared that I was going up there (2) and they gave me a balloon (3) and I went to um Toys "R" Us (4) and gave me a toy but I never. . . . (5) I uh I just broke my leg and I just fall down on my bike because I got hurt and (6) my bandaids on me. . . . (7) put their off and I jumped out of my bike and (8) I . . . I flied and then I jumped down.

E: You jumped down?

R: (9) Uhuh, on the grass. . . . (10) and I um our grandma um she died. (11) She um she was getting older (12) Our grandma and she died and the uh funeral . . . (13) My ma and dad went to the funeral and then Aunt Cindy was there too (14) and we uh they um uh everybody was sad that um uh that died . . . (15) and on my birthday I went on my bike and I uh um. . . . (16) I just jump on my bike and I just balance on my. . . . (17) and I did it with uh I did do it with only my hands. (18) I didn't do it without my hands and I uh um one hand too.

Topic Maintenance: Inappropriate. Several topics are intermingled, such as hospital activities, bike riding, and events pertaining to the grandmother.

Event Sequencing: Inappropriate. This sample represents a leapfrogging structure in which events are not presented chronologically. The following events are presented achronologically: broken leg, death of grandmother, and bike ride.

Informativeness: Inappropriate. There is insufficient information for the listener to know what happened to the child's leg; elaboration is reduced; evaluation (utterances 1, 4, 5, etc.) and action (utterances 1, 2, 4, etc.) are well represented, while description is minimal.

Referencing: Variable. Some pronoun identities are specified (utterances 10, 11, 14); some are understood by the context (*they* in utterances 1 and 2), some are unspecified (*there* in utterance 1, *their* in utterance 7) and some are even more vague (*it* in utterances 17 and 18).

Conjunctive Cohesion: Variable. Appropriate semantic cohesion is evident in coordination (utterances 1, 2, 3, etc.), temporal meaning (utterance 8), causality (utterance 1); two violations are evident (utterances 5 and 13); appropriate pragmatic use is found in change of focus (utterances 10 and 15).

Fluency: Inappropriate. False starts (utterances 4, 12, 15, etc.), internal corrections (utterances 10 and 14), repetitions (utterances 8, 11, 12), and excessive use of fillers (utterances 10, 14, 15).

Intervention Goals.   In short, this second speaker struggles with all six dimensions of discourse assessed in NAP. Primary clinical goals would be at the macronarrative level of discourse, such as topic maintenance, event sequencing, and informativeness.

Group Profile of Children with Traumatic Brain Injury (TBI)

Following is a summary of the relatively little information that exists about the narration of children with TBI:

Topic Maintenance

Usually appropriate. Chapman and her colleagues (1992) had children and adolescents with varying degrees of TBI engage in a story retelling task. Only subjects with severe injury were impaired in their abilities to present critical story information and delineate episodes in narratives. Jordan, Murdoch, and Buttsworth (1991) did not find differences in the production of story grammar elements when children with TBI were asked to tell a story about a doll.

Event Sequencing

Variable. While this has not been a focus of prior studies, Chapman et al. (1992) found that children with TBI omitted more essential action information than peers with TLD. On the other hand, Biddle, McCabe, and Bliss (1996) did not find much evidence of disturbed event sequencing compared to individuals with TLD.

Informativeness

Inappropriate. Although children and adults with TBI sometimes produce just as many narrative propositions as peers with TLD (Biddle, McCabe, & Bliss, 1996), they tend to do this by repeating significantly more propositions and by omitting much information that a listener would need to infer in order to make sense of their narrative. That is, they have very inefficient narration. Even more than adults with TBI, children with TBI omit substantial amounts of critical information.

Referencing

Inappropriate. Part of the substantial listener burden for children with TBI that was documented by Biddle, McCabe, and Bliss (1996) was due to problematic referencing.

Conjunctive Cohesion

Appropriate. Jordan, Murdoch, and Buttsworth (1991) did not find differences between children with and without TBI in cohesion in their storytelling task.

Fluency

Inappropriate. In narratives of personal experience, children with TBI were vastly more dysfluent than adults with TBI or typical controls of any age (Biddle, McCabe, & Bliss, 1996).

Consider a sample narrative from a child with TBI, followed by a NAP of that narrative:

> *Example from 7-year-, 4-month-old girl with traumatic brain injury (TBI)*
> *(from Biddle, McCabe, & Bliss, 1996)*
> E: Did you ever get stung by a bee?
> T: (1) Umm, I, once, there was a, we went. (2) There was a for. (3) There was this umm fort. (4) A tree fell down. (5) And there was dirt, all kinds of stuff there. (6) it was our fort. (7) And one day, I have a friend named Jude. (8) She's umm grown up. (9) She has a kid. (10) She has a cat named Gus, a kitten. (11) It's so cute. (12) But once, when she didn't have that kitten, one day, me, my brother, my cousin Matt, and her, and my dad, and one of his friends, went into the woods to see the fort, to show her. (13) And we went up there. (14) I stepped on a bee's nest. (15) And they chased us all the way back. (16) And I got stung, (17) and my cousin Matt got stung in one of the private parts. (18) And ummm I had a bite right here (points), right here (points), right there (points), and ummm one on my cheek. (19) And right here. (20) And when I um went over, when we got back to my friend Jude's house, in her bathroom she had this clean kind of stuff. (21) And I put it on me. (22) She put it on me right here (points). (23) But umm, I had to go to the bathroom to put it on, you know. (24) It hurt! (25) And my brother Jason he got stung once. (26) He got stung I think three right here (points). (27) I remember where I got stung, (28) but I don't remember where Jason got stung. (29) My friend Jude didn't even get stung. (30) She ran so fast that she didn't even get stung. (31) The bees chased us, (32) and I looked back. (33) And there was one right in front of my face. (34) That's when I got stung here (points). (35) There was like two hanging around my legs. (36) I was running and trying to get them off me. (37) They both went, "Bzzzz." (38) It hurt! (39) I was crying my head off.

Topic Maintenance: Appropriate. There is some tangential information about Jude (she has a kid and a kitten) at the outset of the narrative, but it serves as a character sketch that enriches the story.

Event Sequencing: Variable. Most of the narrative consists of chronologically sequenced events, although utterances 31–39 constitute a whole chunk of chronologically sequenced events that would more appropriately have been told before or after utterance 16. While individuals without TBI also do this sort of recycling on occasion, they would usually signal it in some way.

Informativeness: Appropriate. Enough information is presented for the listener to understand the narrative, which is not typical of individuals with TBI The narrative is sufficiently elaborated. There is adequate description (e.g., utterances 5–10), action (e.g., utterances 12–16), and evaluation (e.g., utterances 11, 24, 38).

Referencing: Variable. While we do not know to whom *we* (utterance 1) or *our* (utterance 6) refer, she does introduce Jude and "my cousin Matt" and "my brother Jason" and subsequently refer to them with pronouns.

Conjunctive Cohesion: Variable. The speaker only uses *and* and *but* and could use practice with *then, because,* and *so.* However, the two conjunctions she uses serve numerous purposes. *And* is used semantically to represent coordination (e.g., 5, 7, 13, etc.), temporal sequence (utterance 32), and causality (e.g., 15–19). *But* denotes a semantically adversative relationship (28), as well as, pragmatically, a change of topic (12 and 23).

Fluency: Inappropriate. As is typical of individuals with TBI, this girl struggles with numerous false starts (e.g., utterances 1, 2, 7, 20), corrections (e.g., 22 corrects 21, 26 corrects 25) and repetitions (e.g., utterances 13 and 18 are repetitious in themselves or of prior material).

Intervention Goals.   For full information regarding intervention strategies with children, see Chapter 8. Meanwhile, here and throughout chapters prior to Chapter 8, we will provide an outline of *what* needs to be done with specific children. Again, Chapter 8 will provide the *how-to* of accomplishing that. The intervention goal of most importance here is to increase self-monitoring of narrative discourse. Individuals with TBI frequently have impairments in executive functions. This deficit results in discourse that does not appear to be organized or planned. This speaker needs to learn to produce a concise narrative that does not appear to be "rambling" and to monitor herself for departures from relevant information. Excessive dysfluencies also reflect planning deficiencies. With increased self-monitoring, we would expect improvements in conciseness and fluency.

Group Profile of Children with Early Corrective Heart Surgery (ECHS)

Lowry Hemphill and David Bellinger and their collaborators have assessed the narrative development of children who are at risk for discourse problems because of histories of early corrective heart surgery at ages 4 and 8 (Hemphill, Uccelli, Willenberg, & Bellinger, 2001; Hemphill, Uccelli, Winner, & Chang, 2002; Ovadia, Hemphill, Winner, & Bellinger, 2000). The following information is based upon their work. Children with ECHS who were studied were born with a common birth defect—transposition of the great arteries—that requires surgery in infancy. Children with histories of such early corrective heart surgery (ECHS) for transposition of the great arteries rarely experience later heart problems, but the surgery puts them at risk for delays in a range of areas, including language development. Lack of oxygen and trauma associated with circulatory arrest and cardiopulmonary bypass put cognitive, motor, and language functions at risk.

Topic Maintenance

Children with ECHS are able to sustain talk on topics initiated by their parents or themselves over several turns, but show difficulty in sustaining a narrative frame. Such children often fall back upon repetition of themselves and others to extend narrative sequences.

Event Sequencing

Children with ECHS do not characteristically narrate events out of logical or temporal sequence. However, their sparse and unelaborated reporting of events (see "Informativenesss") can result in narratives that are missing a key happening.

Informativeness

Children with ECHS show clear difficulty with narrative informativeness. At both ages 4 and 8 years, their personal narratives were much shorter than those of comparison children, averaging less than half the length of comparison children's. Twelve of the seventy-six children with ECHS assessed at age 4 were not able to produce narrative talk at all in response to multiple prompts for a narrative of personal experience. While at age 8 all children with ECHS were able to produce some narrative talk concerning several personal experiences, their narratives on average were impoverished in the reporting of events, orientation, and evaluation—all three critical constituents of narrative. In these critical respects, 8-year-old children with ECHS more resembled typically developing 4-year-olds. At both 4 and 8 years, the largest gaps between the narrative performance of children with ECHS and children with TLD are evident in the provision of orientation, character intentions, and internal emotional states.

Referencing

Referencing nouns appears to be a strength of children with ECHS.

Conjunctive Cohesion

Children with ECHS include fewer causal conjunctions in their narratives than typically developing children at ages 4 and 8 years. Such children tend to rely too much on all-purpose connectives such as *and*.

Fluency

Many children with ECHS show problems with fluency at age 4. Such problems, often involving articulation difficulty, are much less evident at age 8.

Example Narratives from Children with Other Disorders

Due to a lack of systematic relevant research, there is far less information available on the narratives of children who exhibit other disorders. However, we do have some examples of children with various disorders, which follow, along with NAPs of those narratives.

Example from 8-year-old girl with hearing impairment (from our collection)
(1) Only my dad [has been in an accident]. (2) My dad had a accident, when, um . . . a bump he head. (3) It was bleeding. (4) His arm split SHHHH (gestures where the father's arm was cut). (5) Hurt his head in the back. (6) Then he hit his arm on the um on the seat (7) and it was really, really hard. (8) And that how, um, Dad came home with the hospital. (9) then we came home, (10) and I went to my bedroom and cried (11) and Andrew and Mallerie were just sitting there watching a movie. (12) And my mommy um could let me come in and in Dad's room and sit on his lap, my dad's lap. (13) It make me pretty sad right now.

Topic Maintenance: Appropriate. All the utterances seem to relate to her dad's accident.

Event Sequencing: Appropriate. Events are presented in chronological order.

Informativeness: Inappropriate. There is not enough information presented to make sense of the accident, how the child's dad got from the accident to the hospital, or the homecoming. Why does the child mention Andrew and Mallerie's watching a movie and how does this relate to the father's homecoming? There is almost no true description, although there is some evaluative description (3, 4, 5, 7) and some pure evaluation (13). There is plenty of action (e.g., 6, 8, 9, 10).

Referencing: Variable. There is some appropriate use of pronouns such as *he* and *his* to refer to her father (4, 5, 6, etc.). However, *it* is unspecified (7), *he* is used instead of *his* (2), and we can only guess that Andrew and Mallerie are siblings. The speaker aptly monitors herself on this dimension (12), which is a good sign.

Conjunctive Cohesion: Variable. The discourse is choppy partly because of few conjunctions. Such relatively noncohesive presentation is characteristic of individuals with hearing or language impairment. However, the speaker uses *and* for coordination (7, 11) and temporal sequencing (8, 10, 12). *Then* is also used plausibly for temporal sequencing (6, 9). The speaker does not use *but, because,* or *so,* nor are any conjunctions used for pragmatic purposes.

Fluency: Inappropriate. There are several fillers (6, 8, 12) and internal corrections (12), which are considerable in this brief narrative.

Intervention Goals.   The goals for this speaker are to increase informativeness and referencing. The clinician can guide the child in making her narrative more informative by using contingent queries (see Chapter 8 for more detail regarding this procedure; in this case contingent queries might include, "So you and your family had to take your dad to the hospital? What happened there?").

Although not a narrative concern per se, the child also has problems with using prepositions and verbs grammatically (e.g., *with* is used instead of *from* in utterance 8; *could let* is used instead of simply *let* in utterance 12). Such difficulties found in narrative need to be noted but should be distinguished from narrative problems.

Example from 12-year-old boy with mental retardation (from our files)
Note that when the clinician departs from protocol to make an exclamation, she influences the story line; the child responds, "That's what the bus driver said." This kind of influence detracts from our ability to know what the child is inclined to do on his own, though it would be appropriate in therapy.

> (1) Oh I seen, I seen two cars crashed up (2) but I didn't see it. (3) One of the buses got in a accident. (4) Well, what happened is, I guess, she was driving. (5) She was turning. (6) She hit the curb. (7) I guess hit the tree then hit the fence and ran into a house. (Clinician: Wow!) (8) That's what the bus driver said. (9) And I guess she got a new bus, (10) and plus when I was going somewhere, me, my brother, and my mom were going somewhere, we seen two cars in a parking crashed up. (11) I don't know how it happened, just seen it. (12) It's crashed up.

Topic Maintenance: Appropriate. The speaker talks about two car accidents he either heard about or saw.

Event Sequencing: Appropriate. Events are in chronological order.

Informativeness: Inappropriate. The speaker omits subjects (7), but this could be a colloquial or personal style. The narrative needs elaboration in general; unless the speaker shows himself capable of telling more elaborate narratives on other topics, such a lack of elaboration is an important impairment. There is action information (3, 5, 6, 7, etc.). There is only limited description of "crashed-up" (10, 12). There is no evaluation.

Referencing: Variable. Linguistic evidence exists that the speaker is from a lower socioeconomic group in his use of the construction "I seen." The reason that this is probably a feature of low socioeconomic dialect rather than retardation is that elsewhere in this same sample, the child demonstrates an ability to use the copula/auxiliary construction ("was driving") and complex sentences (e.g., 10). As was mentioned earlier regarding low SES, one might reasonably expect an implicit style of referencing, which is what one in fact finds here: *it* is used ambiguously (2, 12); *she* is used when the referent had previously been given as "One of the buses" only. While the speaker aptly refers to "a house" when it is first introduced, he uses a more colloquial "the curb" the first time that is introduced. In short, given the many other problems this speaker faces, his habits in this area might well be socioeconomic ones and not ones to be addressed in therapy, especially given his critical problem with informativeness.

Conjunctive Cohesion: Appropriate. Speaker uses *and, but,* and *then* to indicate, respectively, coordination, adversative, and temporal relationships between utterances. *And* (9) is used for temporal relationship, and *and plus* (10) is used pragmatically to indicate the commencement of a new narrative.

Fluency: Appropriate, despite one internal correction (10).

Intervention Goals.   This speaker primarily needs to elaborate his narrative. Listeners need more specific information to understand the message and more details to become engaged by it.

Example from a 9-year-, 5-month-old boy with attention deficit hyperactivity disorder (ADHD) (from our files)
Adult: What happened when you went to the hospital when your dog bit you?

Child: (1) Well, he was chewing up something (2) and I did not like it. (3) But you know what? (4) He was being such a . . . such a . . . (5) He was being so sick . . . (6) He was just chewing it up, sucking. (7) I got mad at him (8) and . . . and . . . then I. . . . just I just tried to spank him (9) and he really didn't notice who was behind him and (10) and I and I was playing Nintendo, you know . . . (11) but then, well I was fixin' to jump so he could just scratch the table . . . (12) but . . . but . . . um . . . before I could even jump, he bit me right on my lip, right here. (13) Can you see the scar here still? (14) But, you know what? (15) When I had to get the stitches out . . . (16) You wanna know about the really stupid lady? (17) I hope she got fired. (18) You know why? (19) She was so stupid (20) You know what she did? (21) Well you see umm . . . umm (22) Well not the stupid lady. (23) These people that were trying to take out my stitches . . . (24) They were umm . . . umm . . . (25) No matter how strong they are . . . (26) They're so stupid . . . (27) 'Cause they just . . . , you know . . . (28) You should get the point. (29) But, you know what? (30) You know how they were taking my stitches out? (31) They just like, when they put them it. (32) Uhmm, even when they, you know . . . they were just pull them all up like that and then like that (gestures to indicate a pulling direction) (33) and then like that (more pulling gestures) or something (34) and then I just couldn't hold still (35) uum . . . so then they get this one dopey lady to come hold me down (36) and then . . . um, mm she hold me down so hard. . . . (37) um . . . when I got out of there in the park . . . in the parking lot there was. . . . (38) I had this big bruise on my cheek. (39) She grabbed me that hard.

Topic Maintenance: Variable. While all the utterances pertain to the dog bite and its consequences, the narrative takes a strange turn at utterances 21–22. We do not know why, now that the narrator has piqued our curiosity about "the stupid lady," he departs to a discussion of the people who "were trying to take out" his stitches.

Event Sequencing: Appropriate. All events are sequenced chronologically.

Informativeness: Variable. We have enough specific facts, as well as ample elaboration. There are abundant references to actions (1, 8, 9, etc.), evaluation (2, 5, 7, 17, etc.), though virtually no pure description per se. The narrator also has informativeness problems that he himself indicates (28); when he says, "You should get the point," we do not.

Referencing: Variable. The interviewer establishes reference to the main actor of the piece—the narrator's dog. The narrator does introduce one other character (16): "You wanna know about the really stupid lady?" However, this is not as helpful as calling the person a nurse (note that "lab technician" would be more applicable, but unlikely even from a child of 9 with TLD). Other vague references include *it* in 2, "one dopey lady" in 35.

Conjunctive Cohesion: Appropriate. The narrator uses *and, but, and then, but then, but before,* and *so* appropriately and abundantly (see utterances 2, 3, 8, 9, 10, 11, 12, 14, 33, 35, etc.) to refer to coordination (2, etc.), temporal sequence (8), causality (35), and adversative (12) relations. There is a pragmatic use of *but* in utterance 11 to refer to a change of focus.

Fluency: Variable. There are a few filled pauses (21, 36) that are common even in the speech of children with TLD. However, there are several abandoned sentences (15, 21, 24, 27) that indicate problems sustaining focus in discourse.

Intervention Goals.   Initially, topic maintenance and informativeness should be targeted. While the speaker shows strengths in these dimensions, he needs to structure a more coherent narrative that adheres more closely to topic maintenance constraints and that provides sufficient information to the listener. These goals will be accomplished through increased self-monitoring, which can be achieved by repeatedly drawing the child's attention to his productions. Increased referencing will likely occur with improvements in the two general areas of discourse coherence.

Example from 16-year-old boy with autism (from our files)
E: My sister was on a swing and she fell off and broke her wrist. Have you ever broken your arm?

J: (1) Yeah.

E: What happened?

J: (2) I broke the wrist on his back. (3) I got throat and the stomach and that boy says, "I got the stomach ache" (4) and the man. . . . and they got. . . . (5) I said, "I hurt my wrist" and umm the man is umm he's a person (6) The man is umm he's a and the man is umm. . . . (7) He got arrested and umm the man is got a chest with a body over (8) and the man is uh person of the man of God.

Topic Maintenance: Inappropriate. The speaker does not maintain a topic; extraneous events are intertwined in his discourse. While some of the topics appear to be associated with pain, the listener cannot discern any unifying topic.

Event Sequencing: Inappropriate. The events are not sequenced in an identifiable pattern.

Informativeness: Inappropriate. The narrative is not explicit enough for the listener to make sense of the story. There is insufficient information and lack of elaboration. There are limited descriptions, actions, and evaluations.

Referencing: Inappropriate. The pronouns *his* (utterance 2) and *they* (utterance 4) are not specified. The identity of "that boy" (utterance 3) and "the man" (utterance 4, 5, 6, etc.) are not provided.

Conjunctive Cohesion: Inappropriate. The conjunction *and* is used to connect seemingly unrelated events (utterance 3, 5, 6 etc.).

Fluency: Inappropriate. False starts (utterances 4, 6), repetitions (utterances 6, 8), and fillers (utterances 5, 6, etc.) are abundant.

Intervention Goals. This speaker is unable to construct a coherent narrative because all of the discourse dimensions are severely compromised. This narrator needs extensive assistance with narrative discourse. Scriptal or procedural discourse may be used as an initial step towards extended discourse. This child needs structured discourse tasks before he can attempt more unstructured dialogues. The initial focus would be on topic maintenance and event sequencing. Modeling would be crucial. With success, less structured forms of discourse could be elicited.

This narrative provides a contrast with the previous samples. While we can understand the other impaired narratives even though there were problems with discourse coherence, we cannot understand this narrative at all even with a great deal of listener interpretation. The NAP permits this type of detailed, contrastive analysis, although we cannot use it to make a differential diagnosis among disorders.

Assessment Considerations

Topic Maintenance

European North American children are expected to maintain topic by the time they enter school (Brinton & Fujiki, 1984; Ervin-Tripp, 1979; Foster, 1986). Language-impaired children frequently provide extraneous or tangential information in their narratives. An inability to maintain a topic should be considered to be a sign of impairment when exhibited by children 7 years and older.

Event Sequencing

Leapfrogging narratives, as was mentioned at the outset of this chapter, are those in which events are not sequenced chronologically and omit crucial information. Such leapfrog narratives are not to be expected from ENA children over the age of 4 years, so this pattern would be a strong sign of impairment in school-aged children.

Informativeness

Detailed narratives are a hallmark of the narratives from ENA children with typical language development. There are times, however, when a child is reticent to speak and may only provide a brief narrative, perhaps due to shyness, unfamiliarity with the topic, lack of attention, or uncooperativeness. A child exhibiting these factors needs to be distinguished from a child who truly cannot produce an informative narrative. A child with a language impairment will generally construct a short and unelaborated narrative, perhaps omitting critical elements. Narratives of school-aged children that do not inform the listener of salient details are considered deficient.

Referencing

Judgments of referencing need to be considered with regard to socioeconomic status. Individuals from low-income backgrounds frequently use unspecified pronouns (Hemphill, 1989). The judgment of typical or impaired referencing depends upon the amount of unspecified referents, the degree to which the referent can be retrieved by the context, or the facility the speaker has to supply the appropriate reference when asked. A speaker who consistently does not appropriately identify pronouns, regardless of SES, would be suspected of impaired referencing. If the listener cannot retrieve any referents in a narrative, an impairment would be suggested because the speaker has provided no background information that is needed to understand a message. In addition, consistent use of vague vocabulary may suggest a word retrieval deficit.

Conjunctive Cohesion

Conjunctions are expected in the narratives of ENA children, and more often mark semantic links than pragmatic ones (Peterson & McCabe, 1991). Typically, the coordinating conjunction *and* is most prevalent in narratives followed by the temporal link *and then* (Peterson & McCabe, 1991). An abundance of these conjunctions does not represent disordered use, despite the fact that teachers often encourage children to omit such conjunctions in their written compositions. Instead, impaired usage is signaled by the absence of conjunctions or, less likely, their frequent semantic misuse (particularly the inappropriate use of causality). However, this type of error rarely occurred in the narratives of children with language impairments that we have collected.

Fluency

Fluent speech production is generally expected from children and adults. Dysfluencies may occur that do not represent a disorder, such as when a speaker hesitates and searches for appropriate wording or concepts to express thoughts. Children frequently overuse the filler *like,* which does not represent a disorder, although it is annoying to many adults. As we noted before, dysfluencies in preschool children tend to increase, while they decrease thereafter in children with typical language development. Dysfluencies that are frequent enough to stop the flow of discourse are considered to be an impairment.

Intervention Considerations

As with any group, narrative assessment offers guidelines for intervention. The focus of remediation should be on the most noticeable and critical aspects of discourse. A form of triage can be performed in which the more minor aspects of discourse, such as conjunctions, should receive less and less immediate attention than the more critical aspects, such as topic maintenance and informativeness. That is, a child who is impaired can produce a narrative without conjunctions that manages nonetheless to convey information: "I ran outside. I stepped on a bee. I got stung." However, a child cannot give conjunctions with an impoverished narrative and communicate much of anything: "And thing. But because it did."

ENA children who do not maintain event sequencing, which is highly valued in their culture, need to learn to do so. They need to be able to structure their narratives around a central topic and to provide critical information. Modeling short structured narratives as an initial step with gradual reduction of structure is advised. Specific techniques for intervention are presented in Chapter 8.

Individual discourse dimensions may need initial focus or can be treated in conjunction with other aspects. For example, referencing can be treated as a separate entity while event sequencing and informativeness may be treated together. In our experience with impaired narration, deficits in the latter two dimensions frequently co-occur. By focusing on event sequencing and informativeness, in other words, professionals can broaden their scope of intervention.

Professionals can use contingent queries in order to enable a child to appropriately use various discourse dimensions (Bliss, 1993). For example, clarifying questions (e.g., "Where did you go? What happened?"; see Chapter 8 for more detail) can indicate to a child that a narrative was not explicit enough, a topic was not maintained or inappropriate referencing was used. Verbal redirection (Lucas, 1980) as well as leading questions, prompts, and answers in discourse-based feedback will assist narrative development. For children with sufficient metapragmatic and metalinguistic abilities, narratives can be analyzed, segmented, and reconstructed to identify specific narrative components and discourse deficits (Naremore, Densmore, & Harman, 1995).

Another strategy that is useful in increasing narrative length and content is scaffolding. Professionals can encourage caregivers to build on their child's utterances in order to assist them in producing longer and more informative messages

(Norris & Hoffman, 1993). Scaffolding can be implemented most successfully with preschool children.

Additional procedures that are designed to foster the use of narrative structure and the six dimensions of NAP will be presented in the chapter on intervention (Chapter 8).

4

African American Children[1]

with Tempii Champion
and Karen Mainess

Expected Features of Narration: African American Children

- A focus on the importance of telling a good story, often by embellishing the facts with the use of metaphors, jokes, slang, exaggeration, refrains, and other classic rhetorical devices.
- Occasional combination of several or even numerous experiences into a single narrative.
- Preference for lengthy narratives.
- Occasional production of a performative (sometimes called topic-associating) narrative that combines several thematically related experiences, each of which is unified by tempo and/or tone.

—adapted from Champion, 1998

---

[1]African American English (AAE) dialectical features are included when children used them. Smitherman (1977) and Labov (1972) provide abundant evidence of the rule-governed nature of AAE.

Example Narratives from Children with Typical Language Development

The development of narration in this community is complex and diverse, with many variations due to geography, class, gender, individual, and many other factors. Nonetheless, some broad patterns may be noted.

Preschool oral narrative—4-year-old African American boy (from our files)
Ben: You know what? I was in a surfing board?

Adult visitor: Right.

Ben: It was a blue surfing board, and I turned over in deep water? I can swim, and Daddy didn't see, and he saw the board, and you know what? And I got in, when I got in, I turned it out. So I had to hold my nose. I can't I can't, I was tryin' to go like that, when I was trying do go over to the rock. When Dad comes in here, he says, "Why are you sittin' down? How'd you get in there? Thought you'd swim under the waterfall? I mean, I thought you went through the cave way and jumped over the table under the sea. Like Superman!"

Father: You got a good one [story] tonight!

Key points about this narrative include:

- This is a good narrative from a preschool child. All of the propositions are about one topic, swimming in a fancy hotel pool with a waterfall.
- The narrative is lengthy for a child his age, and for that reason he does not tell all the events that he would were he a year or two older. This relative lack of clarity should not be mistaken as deficient. Peterson and McCabe (1983) found that such leapfrogging narratives were the most common structure to be found among the longest narratives of European North American preschool children with typical language development. Champion (1998) found that narratives in some ways resembling leapfrog structure were told by older African American children and were better understood as "performative" narratives.

Topic-centered narrative—5-year-old African American preschool child (from our files: African American preschool-aged children from a Head Start program were asked to tell a story about something that they did or anything else that they wanted to do)
I broke my leg. And I had to go to the doctor. And they gave me a shot. And I didn't even cry. And I got a sticker. And I went home.

Key points about this narrative include:

- Every clause is related to a single topic of breaking a leg (singularity of theme).
- A linear sequence (organization) of events is narrated in the order in which the events occurred.
- There is complicating action (going to the doctor, getting a shot) and an evaluative high point ("I didn't even cry").

- Resolution is provided: "And I went home."
- The narrator includes much thematic cohesion in the form of repetition of key lexical items (e.g., five propositions start with "I")

Topic-associating or performative narration—5-year-old African American preschool child (from our files)

My friend, Hershel and David (spilled something). They work with Daddy. And then they spilled . . . they spill. Herschel, Herschel spilled milk. David don't spill nothing. Some of my friends get tied up like this (gestures). The shoe kinda like that. Then they fall. Hurt and hurt his head. They had to put a bandage on his head. And then and then he had a puppy, named Roxy. I had a puppy named Roxy. Though, but but he ran away, though. Some dogs run away though.

Some key points about this narrative are:

- Lengthiness characterizes the topic-associating style (Michaels, 1991) found in this narrative.
- Champion (1998) calls this an example of performative narrative structure.
- The narrator includes frequent shifts in time frame, location, and participants but events are organized around the theme of "recent events in the life of people and animals I love."

Topic-centered narrative—6-year-old African American boy (from files of Tempii Champion)

Child: 'Cause, um when we go outside an den when we go far den she gets

Adult: So where are you supposed to stay?

Child: In 'a backyard but we went to go jump off a roof.

Adult: You went to jump off a roof? What happened?

Child: Nothin'.

Adult: Did you jump off the roof?

Child: Yeah!

Adult: Well something happened then! Tell me what happened.

Child: We went um we went to the behind the store. There was just a little roof, an den da roof was up to the ceiling. An' then there was a big snowbank. Almost, actually it was right like (gestures). An' den we jumped down. Dat's all we did. That's that's why my mom got mad at us.

Some key points about this narrative are:

- This is a topic-centered narrative about one time when the narrator was mischievous.
- Because this narrative occurred in the context of an ongoing conversation, the child had probably already identified the "we" of the narrative for the listener; in all likelihood the child and his siblings constituted "we."

- The narrative is a classic in that it builds to a high point ("We jump down") that is clearly evaluated ("That's all we did").
- The resolution of the story is that that incident explains his mother's anger at him.

Performative oral narrative—8-year-old African American girl (collected by Mignonne Pollard, from our files)

We went to the dentist before, and I was gettin' my tooth pulled. And the doc, the dentist said, "Oh, it's not gonna hurt." And he was lying to me. It hurt. It hurted so bad I coulda gone on screamin' even though I think some . . . (I don't know what it was like). I was, in my mouth like, I was like, "Oh that hurt!" He said no, it wouldn't hurt. Cause last time I went to the doctor, I had got this spray. This doctor, he sprayed some spray in my mouth and my tooth appeared in his hand. He put me to sleep, and then, and then I woke up. He used some pliers to take it out, and I didn't know. So I had told my, I asked my sister how did, how did the man take (it out). And so she said, "He used some pliers." I said, "Nah, he used that spray." She said, "Nope he used that spray to put you to sleep, and he used the pliers to take it out." I was, like, "Huh, that's amazin'." I swear to God I was so amazed that, hum . . . It was so amazing, right? That I had to look for myself, and then I asked him too. And he said, "Yes, we, I used some pliers to take out your tooth, and I put you to sleep, an, so you wouldn't know, and that's how I did it." And I was like, "Ooouuu." And then I seen my sister get her tooth pulled. I was like, "Ooouuu" cause he had to put her to sleep to, hmm, to take out her tooth. It was the same day she got her tooth pulled, and I was scared. I was like, "EEEhhhmmm." I had a whole bunch cotton in my mouth, chompin' on it 'cause I had to hold it to, hmm, stop my bleeding. I, one day I was in school. I took out my own tooth. I put some hot water in it the night, the, the night before I went to school. And I was taking a test. And then it came out right when I was takin', when I finished the test. And my teacher asked me, was it bleeding. I said, "No, it's not bleeding, cause I put some hot water on it." And so my cousin, he wanted to take out his tooth, and he didn't know what to do, so I told him. "I'm a Pullin' Teeth Expert. Pull out your own tooth, but if you need somebody to do it, call me, and I'll be over."

This narrative is an example of an engaging account of multiple personal experiences with dentistry that are thematically integrated into one story, the story of a "Pullin' Teeth Expert." It includes many of the characteristics of an excellent narrative; specifically, it meets the standard for oral narration in third grade (see *Speaking and Listening for Preschool through Third Grade*, New Standards Project, 2001 (available from National Council for Education and Economy, *www.ncee.org*):

- The narrator presents several sequences of events in such detail that she makes them quite believable.
- She gives the setting of the story ("We went to the dentist before") and introduces characters (the dentist, her sister, her teacher, her cousin) and objects (the spray, some pliers, cotton).
- She portrays the characters succinctly, but vividly and contrastively, often through quotations of them ("The dentist said, 'Oh, it's not gonna hurt.' And he was lying to me. It hurt"; whereas the narrator's sister is truthful, even

though the narrator challenges her version: "She said, 'He used some pliers.' I said, 'Nah, he used that spray . . .').

- She presents enough detail to sustain listeners' interest ("This doctor, he sprayed some spray in my mouth and my tooth appeared in his hand").
- The narrative contains several sequences of as many as eight events, each sequence one of the thematic episodes (e.g., "One day I was in school. I took out my own tooth. I put some hot water in it the night . . . before I went to school, and I was taking a test. And then it came out right when I finished the test. And my teacher asked me, 'Was it bleeding?' I said, 'No, it's not bleeding because I put some hot water on it' ").
- The narrator embeds sequenced events in ongoing activity ("And I was getting' my tooth pulled").
- While the narrator could have given specific dates about exactly when events occurred, such information would be irrelevant to her story. Rather she gives more appropriate, contextualized information about the timing of events ("It was the same day she got her tooth pulled"; tooth "came out right when I . . . finished the test").
- She pays much attention to the motivation of her characters (The dentist "had to put her (sister) to sleep to take out her tooth"; the narrator chews on cotton to stop her bleeding).
- The narrative contains lively subjective commentary that is concentrated in spots ("And I was scared. I was like, 'EEEhhhmmm. I had a whole bunch cotton in my mouth, chompin' on it cause I had to hold it to stop my bleeding") and clearly conveys to the listener the meaning of the various events narrated and the reason the narrator found these events compelling enough to tell.
- She mentions her cousin's goal ("he wanted to take out his tooth") and gives him the means to achieve it.
- The resolving coda is an outstanding one: "I'm a Pullin' Teeth Expert. Pull out your own tooth. But if you need somebody to do it, call me and I'll be over."

Topic-centered narrative from a 10-year-old girl with typical language development (from files of Tempii Champion)
Adult: Have you ever been a hero?

Child: Yes I been a hero to my brother, my brother an' my friends. Well I was ridin' my bike da street, and um, an my friend who was goin real fast cause I was taggin' 'er. An I da thing and had a race to see who' d won. An I was an I an I was tweeny seconds cause I had had had big gear. An' I zoomin' an' she comin' slow. I woulda had forty seconds. I was countin' myself an she counts so she says twenty seconds. An' I said your turn. I had a timer watch. An' she was racing down da street. An' she run she was zoomin on da bike. She's use my bike. She didn know how da gear. An' I said do you know how? An' she says she did 'cause she always like to be you know know-it-all. An' I said don' say you know if you don'. She said 'I know.' An' den a little girl was walkin' across da street an comin across da street. An' she'd been runnin'. She was goin' real fast. An I an I said her name was Kim. An' I said, "Watch out! Watch out!" An' she didn' hear me cause she had a walkman on. An I an I run as fas' I could. An I just in time before she wa' close to her I pushed her aside. An an den um an den she an den den um she an I pushed her aside. An I moved aside so she wouldn' t hit her. An den den she said, "Whe where was dat little girl at?" An I said, "She came across da street an you almos' hit her. An she got she pick da little girl up. She said sorry. An da las thing dat happened was she jus' threw my bike in da road. An now I need a nother one. I have a kickstand, but she didn' put it down. She jus threw it. I said da bike—I said "Da little girl was importan', but you didn't have throw it down. An' I saved 'er. You were gonna hit 'er." And dat's all.

Key points about this narrative include:

- This is an example of what Champion (1998) called Moral Centered Structure, defined as a story in which the narrator embeds a lesson for the audience— in this case about the inevitable downfall of know-it-alls.
- It is organized around the high-point event of pushing the little girl out of harm's way, an event that is reiterated evaluatively three times. Such repetition has been termed a form of parallelism, a discourse tactic typical of African American communication style (Foster, 1995). Parallelism signals what content is important across utterances, and is often found in African American children's narration (Champion, Katz, Muldrow, & Dail, 1999).

Example of narration from a 12-year-old girl, middle socioeconomic status
(from the files of Karen Mainess)
Oh yeaah. I was talking to this boy that my friend really, really, really liked. She was like in love with him. And like, they're like friends. But he treats her really bad, and she cries all the time about it. So I talked to him and like saying, "You should be nicer to her" all of that stuff. And then, cause he's just really a jerk (laugh). It's funny sometimes and then he like, I remember this time I was talking about her to him. Like how, I was like telling him "be nicer to her because when you don't and she starts crying, she calls me up crying, saying how much she hates you," and stuff like that. And then she was like right behind me when I was saying it. (laughs). And I was laughing. She was laughing too. She was like, "Bea!" And I just ran into my class. I was laughing though.

Among the most important features of this narrative are:

- This is another topic-centered narrative, with a clear high point ("she was like right behind me when I was saying it" . . . laughs are a clear evaluative device).
- The narrative is resolved by laughter and by the narrator telling how she ran into her class.

Typical Narrative Development

Topic Maintenance

The ability to link sentences into narrative discourse is in place by the time children are in preschool, as the previous examples demonstrate. However, African American children differ from European North American children in that the African

American culture offers at least two distinct ways of developing a narrative topic. Several examples are what has been termed topic-centered narration (Michaels, 1991), the most common type of oral personal narration from African American (Champion, Seymour, & Camarata, 1995; Hyon & Sulzby, 1994) and European North American children (Peterson & McCabe, 1983). Such narration gives details of a single incident that happened one particular time in one particular place, its beginning, middle, and end.

The third and fifth examples, however, demonstrate an alternative type of topic maintenance, in which a variety of incidents that happened at different times and places, often to different protagonists, are linked thematically (Michaels, 1991). Sometimes children will spell out the theme, such as one girl does ("I'm a Pullin' Teeth Expert"), that unifies all the experiences. At other times, the audience is expected to infer that theme, such as in the third example above, which is roughly, "what has been going on recently in my life with people and animals I love."

Topic-associating narratives are usually longer than topic-centered ones (Michaels, 1991) and may occur more often when children are performing for a crowd of their peers, such as during a sharing time event at school, than in personal conversations. Champion, Seymour, and Camarata (1995) found that two-thirds of the narratives told by 6- to 10-year-old African American children in one-on-one conversations with an adult were topic-centered narratives that began with orientation, proceeded with a series of events that culminated in a high point, and were then resolved—the kind of narrative commonly told in the same situation by their European North American counterparts. In fact, Champion et al. (1995) found that African American children were more likely to tell such a classic narrative than were European North American children.

At first glance, the performative, or topic-associating, form of narration could be seen as the kind of leapfrogging narrative that preschool European American children tell (Peterson & McCabe, 1983). However, there are substantial differences. Specifically, performative, topic-associating narration thematically combines incidents that happened at different times and places, often to different people, while leapfrogging narration pertains by definition to a single incident that happened at one particular place and time to a particular set of characters but is given in such a way that the narrator jumps around temporally and leaves out key events (see Chapter 3).

Event Sequencing

As should be abundantly clear from all the preceding examples, African American children's narratives are filled with lengthy sequences of events told in the order in which they were likely to have happened. As previously mentioned, to European North American ears, the performative (or topic-associating) style may seem to jump around in time and leave out events—the hallmarks of what Peterson and McCabe (1983) termed "leapfrogging" in their sample of European North American children. In fact, Champion and colleagues (1995) found a small number of leapfrogging narratives told by children 6 to 10 years old, which, again, are better understood as performative narratives, readily understood in light of prosody and valued within the community for their length. Furthermore, we would argue that assembling several sets of events (each separate set chronologically ordered, as in the Pullin' Teeth example) into a thematically linked story is a very different enterprise from telling a disjointed sequence.

Informativeness

Police officer's needs: Do you understand the incident the speaker is trying to relate? All three types of informativeness are valued within African American culture. Individuals are expected to provide enough information about an incident for their listeners to understand what is going on. With performative or topic-associating narration, the audience understands that the point of the narrative is not to detail events that happened on one particular occasion, but rather to develop a theme.

Teacher's goals: Did the speaker give ample detail or just the bare bones of the incident? The kind of informativeness that involves elaboration is especially valued in the African American community. Lengthy narratives are expected and enjoyed. In fact, from a young age, children are encouraged to elaborate, using poetic license to develop an entertaining, satisfying story even if a particular experience was a bit lackluster. This strong preference for elaboration has sometimes been misunderstood as "lying" or "rambling" by European North American peers (Craddock-Willis & McCabe, 1996) and teachers (Michaels, 1991). African American adults, however, understand and appreciate such verbal accomplishments (Michaels, 1991).

A preference for narrative elaboration in African American children also depends to some extent on gender and socioeconomic class (SES) (Mainess, Champion, & McCabe, 2002). Among 11- and 12-year-old African American children, girls elaborated more than did boys and, surprisingly, low SES background children elaborated more than their middle-class peers.

Chef's ingredients: Are action, orientation, and evaluation present? Several studies (Champion, Seymour, & Camarata, 1995; Champion, 1998, Kernan, 1977; Labov, 1972) of African American children document ample use of all the key ingredients of a narrative—description, evaluation, and action.

Referencing

To our knowledge, there are no studies that directly compare the referencing styles of African American children from lower to those of middle socioeconomic status, though referential strategies used by preadolescent African American speakers have been described (Hyter, 1994). Presumably, a similar pattern to that documented for European North Americans would be discovered, namely that middle-class individuals prefer a more explicit style of reference, while individuals from a lower socioeconomic background prefer to collaborate more with listeners, who are expected to infer the specific referents for many pronouns (Hemphill, 1989). Hyter and Westby (1996) argue that children and adolescents who use such an implicit style should be taught strategies for unambiguous use of pronominal reference.

As is the case for European North American children, young children have vocabularies that are relatively limited compared to their older counterparts, and this means that sometimes they will use a nonspecific pronoun where a specific pronoun would be clearer. Furthermore, when a young child is talking to a person familiar with the events in question, as in the first example in this chapter, the child will be less specific than when speaking with someone unfamiliar with the events. Again, there is nothing specific to the culture about this phenomenon; it has been documented for European North American preschool children as well (Menig-Peterson, 1975).

Conjunctive Cohesion

As the previous examples amply demonstrate, the narratives of African American children with typical language development are rife with conjunctions. Champion (1995) examined the narratives of 6- to 10-year-old children and found that they used numerous conjunctions and that they used them almost always accurately to encode the five major semantic connections between sentences: coordination, causality, antithesis, temporal sequence, and enabling.

Fluency

Again, we know of no specific studies addressing the issue of fluency in African American individuals. However, all of the authors have had extensive experience working with children and adults from this community and with transcripts of their discourse and have found nothing that would indicate a cultural difference with respect to fluency. In other words, in this culture, individuals with typical language development are fluent.

Example Narratives from African American Children with Impaired Discourse

We turn now to examples of children who are struggling with narrative productions. These narratives were elicited by a friendly adult using the same procedure that was used at the outset of this chapter with typically developing children. The samples have been taken from our unpublished collection.

> *Example from 10-year-old African American boy with specific language impairment (SLI)*
> **Adult:** Have you ever broken any bones?
> **Child:** (1) No, no really, but . . . but I got hit by a car once.

Adult: You did? Tell me about it.

Child: (2) I was 5 years old. (3) I had a bike (4) and I had my eyes closed (5) and this car just. . . . boom.

Adult: Oh, what happened?

Child: (6) Uhm, my leg was kind of . . . it . . . no, no blood (7) but it was pretty messed up.

Adult: What happened after that?

Child: (8) And then, like when I fell down, I knocked myself out on my bike.

Adult: Who, what happened next?

Child: (9) And then, then I woke up. (10) I was in a bed.

Topic Maintenance: Appropriate. All the utterances relate to one injury experience in a topic-centered way.

Event Sequencing: Appropriate. The narrator begins with an abstract and proceeds to elaborate the series of events that culminated in his injury in the order they occurred.

Informativeness: Inappropriate. We have the basic facts of the incident reported here, though we would probably benefit from more details. We know his eyes were closed while he was riding and can easily infer that that is the reason for the accident in the narrator's mind, yet we don't know where the accident occurred, for example.

Especially in view of the value placed on elaboration of stories in the African American community, this narrative seems lacking. Why were his eyes closed? Was he going fast or slowly? What kind of car hit him? Did he wake up in a bed at home or in the hospital? Despite the fact that the incident would lend itself to a memorable story, and despite the fact that the narrator is old enough for us to expect a lengthy story from him, this narrator does not go beyond the barest of bones in his telling. The overall development of his narrative is closer to that of the 4- or 6-year-old African American children with typical language at the outset of this chapter than it is to the older children (note the story about a bicycle accident told by a 10-year-old girl with typical language development at the outset of this chapter).

All the major constituents of narrative are included: description ("I was 5 . . . and had a bike"), evaluation ("pretty messed up"), and action ("fell down . . ." "woke up").

Referencing: Appropriate. We understand his use of "this car" (5) to be colloquial. The use of *it* to refer to "leg" (7) is appropriate.

Conjunctive Cohesion: Appropriate. The narrator begins with a pragmatic use of *but* to indicate the opening of a narrative related to but somewhat different from the topic prompted. There are several coordinate uses of *and* to connect sentences about his having a bike and having his eyes closed and the car's appearance. *But* is used correctly to denote antithesis ("no blood . . . but it was pretty messed up"). The narrator accurately uses *when* structure to code the consequences of falling off his bike. Finally, the narrator closes his narrative with *and then* construction, again an accurate temporal connection.

Fluency: Appropriate. There are a couple of repeated words (e.g., *but*) and one abandoned utterance describing his leg, but these are not unusual even for individuals with typical language development.

Intervention Goals.   This speaker needs to construct narratives with more information. The clinician should provide models, prompts, and cues in order to assist the child in providing sufficient information for the listener.

> *Example from 7½-year-old African American boy with hearing impairment (from files of Bliss & McCabe)*
> **Adult:**   (tells story about an argument she had) Have you ever fought with someone? Tell me about it.
> **Child:**   No . . . My sister and my cousin. He break the table dem fight. Cause dem arguing about dem clothes. Dat's her clothes. Dat's dem clothes and den dem say, "Hold up. Come on." (*Narrator gets into a fighting position with both fists up.*) Dem break de table hard. Dem say (narrator slams fist on the table).
> **Adult:**   And the table broke?
> **Child:**   Yeah.
> **Adult:**   And then what happened?
> **Child:**   Den we have to let is outside. Wait for my bi- Michael come, and den he fix it. And now it's little. Dat's it.

Topic Maintenance: Appropriate. All the utterances pertain to a particular fight between the narrator's sister and cousin.

Event Sequencing: Appropriate. The narrator tells a number of events in sequence (the two argue, threaten, break the table, go outside, wait, then the table gets fixed).

Informativeness: Inappropriate. We get a mere skeleton of a story here, only enough for the proverbial "police officer" in us to understand the basic incident.

As for the kind of elaboration teachers endorse and ordinary listeners enjoy—that is missing here. We know nothing about how old the fighters were, what the clothes they were fighting about looked like, or what exactly the fight consisted of beyond the breaking of the table.

The narrator includes actions (argue, threaten, etc.), a bit of evaluation (table is broken "hard"), and a bit of description (at the end, the table is "little"). However, the overall impression is that he uses dramatic gestures to convey the meaning of the events, the high point of the story.

Referencing: Variable. He clearly introduces the two main characters—his sister and his cousin. But we never find out who Michael is. This narrator may have limited vocabulary, as he acts out several events in the story without putting them also into words. Pronunciation of "them" as "dem" may be a function of dialect (Labov, 1972), hearing impairment, or speech delay.

Conjunctive Cohesion: Appropriate. There is correct usage of causal conjunction ("Dem fight . . . cause dem arguing about dem clothes"), of coordination ("and den dem say," "And now it's little"), and temporal conjunction ("Den we have to let . . ."). In general, however, this narrator does not use *and* as frequently as both African American and European North American children with typical language development do. However, this would probably be considered a strength by teachers concerned with public speaking; frequently starting sentences with conjunctions is a common complaint about typically developing children.

Fluency: Appropriate. This child produces no false starts or internal corrections.

Intervention Goals.   This speaker needs to provide more information for the listener. He needs to offer more facts and elaborate on his experiences. A secondary goal would be to develop flexibility in his referencing skills.

> *Example from 9-year-, 2-month-old African American girl with mental retardation (from files of Bliss, Covington, & McCabe)*
> **Adult:**   Whose birthday party did you go to?
>
> **Child:**   S.
>
> **Adult:**   S. Tell me about S's birthday party.
>
> **Child:**   (*Pauses.*) S. Then we went to the skating rink. Then we went by K. We had said, "Hey K, you wanna go to the skating rink?"
>
> **Adult:**   Tell me more about it.
>
> **Child:**   Then we got some cake. Then we got some candy, cool candy.
>
> **Adult:**   And some candy.
>
> **Child:**   Then we went to Granny's. Then we went to family reunion. Then we went to park. Then we went to the Holiday. Then we went to spend the night for a whole week.
>
> **Adult:**   What else?
>
> **Child:**   Then we had fun. Then we went to the skating ring again and again and again.[2]

Topic Maintenance: Appropriate. All the statements seem to be about having fun with family and friends. She begins and ends with reference to the

---

[2]Bliss, L.S., Covington, Z., & McCabe, A. (1999). Assessing the narratives of African American children. *Current Issues in Communication Sciences and Disorders, 26,* 164–165. © American Speech-Language-Hearing Association. Reprinted by permission.

skating rink. While she may be linking incidents that happened at different places and times (we cannot tell whether the family reunion happened on the same day as the child's birthday party) and thus cannot be sure whether this is a topic-centered or a topic-associating narrative; either is acceptable.

Event Sequencing: Appropriate. She tells the events in a plausible order.

Informativeness: Inappropriate. We do not have enough specific information about the incident to determine whether she is talking about one enjoyable time with lots of component parts or several incidents at different times and places, involving different people.

There is not enough specific information, let alone elaboration. This narrative from a 9-year-old is comparable to the 4-year-old samples at the outset of this chapter, not the lengthy engaging type of narrative we would expect from someone of her age and background.

There is virtually no orientation as to where or when anything happened. We know something about a skating rink and, presumably, a Holiday Inn. But description is for the most part missing. The narrative includes some evaluation ("cool candy") and events. However, twelve out of sixteen propositions consist of the formulaic utterances "Then we went" or "Then we got," which is highly unusual for a child of any age or background.

Referencing: Inappropriate. We never really know who *we* is, but it seems to shift in meaning from friends to family without any notice.

Conjunctive Cohesion: Inappropriate. This child begins twelve of sixteen utterances with *then*, in such a way as to make it seem more a protoconjunction than a meaningful marker of specific types of relationships between sentences.

Fluency: Appropriate.

Intervention Goals.   This child needs to provide more information and elaborate on the events in a narrative. She also needs to learn to provide orientation and descriptive information and to vary sentence structure.

Assessment Considerations

African American children are quite diverse. It is critical for professionals to gather background information about a speaker's cultural communicative style. The models that are used in the home also need to be identified. The most important aspect of assessment is for adults to avoid prejudging children. What is critical here is the specific language experiences of the child. That is, even European North American children who primarily live among and interact with speakers of African American English vernacular should be evaluated using the guidelines in this chapter. Such children, like their African American peers, should not be diagnosed as impaired if they produce a topic-associating form of narrative.

Topic Maintenance

Topic-associating narratives may reflect the communicative style of some members of the African American community. However, previous research has shown that most African American preschool and school-aged children use topic-centered narratives when describing past experiences (Hyon & Sulzby, 1992, 1994; Jones, 1999; Manavathu & Bliss, 1998). Topic-associating styles may be most evident in informal exchanges or in monologues.

Speakers who use African American English (AAE) may either use a topic-centered or topic-associating style. Because a child uses AAE does not mean that a topic-associating style will be evident. Many speakers use AAE features in topic-centered narratives (Champion et al., 1995; Hyon & Sulzby, 1992).

A child may use both a topic-centered and a topic-associating narrative style. Children shift their narrative styles according to different tasks and social situations (Hester, 1996). For this reason, more than one narrative should be elicited in contexts that vary in structure and formality in order to determine a speaker's preferred narrative style and abilities (Hadley, 1998; Hester, 1996; Michaels & Foster, 1985). Different conversational partners should also be used because variations in narratives may be evident with different individuals (Champion et al., 1999). Children with mild impairments may tell embellished or dramatic stories, at least under some circumstances.

Most African American children maintain topic in their personal narratives in a fashion similar to that of European North American children. If digressions occur, the semantic links between topics should be evident to the listener. If questioned about links between events, a child should be able to clarify them for the listener. Signs of impaired topic maintenance are descriptions of unrelated events or presentations of episodes in which semantic associations are not evident to anyone in the child's community. These discourse behaviors suggest that a speaker may not be able to develop a thematically related discourse.

Event Sequencing

Events are chronologically ordered in both topic-centered and topic-associating narratives. Children with typical or impaired language development from African American communities sequence events either in chronological or logical order. When topic-associating narratives are produced, they need to be contrasted with leapfrogging patterns. In the latter, a child does not maintain chronological order, omits critical aspects of a narrative, but describes only *one* occasion. In contrast, topic-associating narratives contain information about *several* occasions within one story. Leapfrogging narratives that are produced by children over 5 years of age would indicate a narrative impairment.

Informativeness

Narratives produced by most African American speakers are informative; they consist of elaborate descriptions with details and evaluations (Champion et al.,

1999; Hyon & Sulzby, 1992, 1994). They are vibrant descriptions of experiences. A speaker from this community who only tells short, unelaborated narratives would be considered impaired.

Referencing

Speakers from lower socioeconomic areas may not specify pronouns. This feature is true of most speakers from lower-class backgrounds and is not unique to African American individuals. Nonstandard pronouns (e.g., *him* for *he*) also do not signal an impairment in narration.

In contrast, two signs of impaired referencing are inappropriate use of pronouns, such as gender violations (e.g., *he* for *she*) and unspecified lexical usage, common in word retrieval deficits.

Conjunctive Cohesion

Conjunctions are common in the narratives of speakers from African American communities. Absence of conjunctions where they are necessary might suggest an inability to link utterances either semantically or pragmatically. Children with language impairment who produce short narratives generally do not use conjunctions.

Fluency

Fluent production is expected from narratives produced by African American speakers. An individual who produces many dysfluencies might also have a word retrieval deficit.

Intervention Considerations

One issue in language remediation is the appropriateness of eliciting a topic-centered style from an African American child who frequently uses a topic-associating structure. One argument against teaching a topic-centered style is that some of the child's peers and members of the community may prefer a topic-associating style.

There are two arguments against this position. First, African American children with typical language development and LI use mostly a topic-centered style in structured discourse contexts (Champion et al., 1999; Hyon & Sulzby, 1992, Labov, 1972; Manavathu & Bliss, 1998). Therefore, this style would not be unfamiliar to a child. Second, many teachers expect a topic-centered narrative style from their students. This style is necessary for success in school, positive evaluations from teachers, and effective communication with teachers who are unaware of the two different narratives styles (Michaels, 1991).

African American children with severe narrative deficits will need to master two-event narratives initially. After they can produce two events, they will need to expand their stories and elaborate them with actions, descriptions, and evaluations. They can accomplish this narrative enhancement in either topic-associating or topic-centered form. Evaluation is a particularly important ingredient since it is prevalent in the narratives of many African American speakers (Labov, 1972).

If a clinician decides to elicit topic-centered narratives, a code switching or bidialectal approach can be used. Terminology, such as "home stories" versus "school stories" can be used (Delpit, 1988). The child can learn to make contrasts between the two contexts and communicative settings and can learn to alternate between the two styles. This approach has been used in eliciting Standard American English forms from speakers who use AAE (Adler, 1979; Campbell, 1996; Delpit, 1988).

One innovative approach to therapy with African American preschool children (aged 3, 4, and 5 years) involved training advanced children in elaborate storybook narration and then pairing these tutors with less advanced children (McGregor, 2000). The children who benefited from such peer tutoring grew in their rate of use of story elements compared to their peers. McGregor (2000) highlighted the benefit of peers for providing culturally congruent therapy in cases where clinicians are not from the same culture as their clients. This approach also seems promising in view of recent calls for adding emergent storybook reading (i.e., retelling familiar storybooks) to language sampling protocols because of its inclusion of written language features (Kaderavek & Sulzby, 2000).

Champion et al. (1999) presented the following recommendations when eliciting narratives from African American children with language disorders: (1) Read and tell stories that are meaningful to the child's culture; (2) encourage adults from the community to tell narratives that describe their own experiences; (3) foster written narratives from children, even preschoolers; (4) encourage children to dictate their stories to adults; and (5) use different and challenging activities to expand print awareness, vocabulary use, and auditory comprehension. Encouraging children to retell familiar storybooks enables them to understand the relationships between oral and written narratives.

In sum, storytelling has always been a vital activity in the African American community (Hurston, 1935/1990). Individuals without the means to tell satisfying stories about their personal experiences should be given every support to acquire these means. At the same time, the rich variety of storytelling enjoyed in the African American community needs to be appreciated and not misdiagnosed as a deficit.

Typical and Disordered Child Narration in Various Cultures

B. Children with English as a Second Language

Following is an overview of issues in bilingualism with some caveats and general advice:

- Second- and third-generation Hispanic Americans have different issues than first-generation individuals. Professionals should never make assumptions about children's cultural background simply by looking at them or their names. We cringe when presented with cases such as the following: Robert's mother is of mixed European North American heritage and his father is second-generation Chinese American. Robert was raised with some very limited exposure to a Chinese dialect, but speaks primarily English. Still, professionals routinely assume from his appearance and last name that he is an "expert" in Chinese. This type of assumption is very misguided. Instead, in conferences with parents, teachers and speech-language pathologists should ask what languages the child speaks and/or understands.
- The complex issues surrounding bilingual education have been thoroughly researched. Still, emotions run high and even a limited review of these issues would be both potentially oversimplified and beyond the scope of this book. What is important for professionals to understand is that numerous studies of many kinds of oral and written language skills document the transfer of language and literacy skills from one language to another (see Cummins, 1991, for review) even in languages with different orthographies, though this diminishes the strength of transference. This means that parental preferences and logistical factors will probably determine which language is used for therapy

with children who lag behind their peers. What is critical is that professionals encourage parents to speak in their native language to their children. The parental input that children require in order to develop enough language to achieve literacy necessitates native proficiency. The only fear for bilingual children is fear of bilingualism itself. If professionals discourage parents from using their strongest language with their children—as they have in this country for years—the children may not receive sufficient linguistic input.

- Variations in bilingual experience are complicated. Children will not become competent bilinguals just by virtue of hearing two languages in various settings. Attention must be paid to how much they hear of both languages and whether they receive the kind of individual, interactive input conducive to language acquisition in both languages (Tabors & Snow, 2001).
- In classrooms that include native English-speaking children as well as those learning English as a second language (ESL), native English-speakers can be enlisted to help their ESL peers learn a variety of English-language skills. Native English-speaking children are seldom recognized for the valuable potential resource they can be in this area. Julie Hirshler (1994) successfully enlisted a number of such children to facilitate the English acquisition of both Spanish- and Kmer-speaking preschool classmates. She made the following recommendations, based on that successful intervention (pp. 235–236):

1. Native English speakers should be trained to interact with second-language learners using strategies such as repetition, restatement, and requests for clarification of their ESL peers. Hirschler reviews the evidence that these strategies have demonstrated benefits for ESL instruction.
2. Language facilitation should be a goal of the class as a group. Focusing on enlisting children who are comfortable in the classroom to help children adjusting to life in a new country with a new language has many potential benefits to the helping children themselves, including promotion of pro-social behavior.
3. Teachers will want to develop all classroom areas with language goals in mind. This is actually a goal of many researchers interested in ensuring that all children—including native speakers who lag behind their peers in terms of language acquisition—develop the oral language skills they will need to successfully acquire literacy skills (Dickinson & Tabors, 2001).
4. Some children are more adept at helping than others. Preschool children learning English as a second language showed a tendency to choose girls as conversational partners rather than play in the same-sex groupings typical of most preschool classrooms. Girls seemed far more skillful at engaging their ESL peers in interaction, and this was much appreciated. What proved disturbing was the tendency of non-English-speaking boys to become isolated in the classroom. Because children learn language through social interaction, and they were receiving very little of this, they were likely to remain isolated unless teachers took steps to include all members of the class in activities and deliberately encourage these boys to interact with peers.

5

Spanish-Speaking American Children

with Nancy Mahecha

Expected Features of Narration: Bilingual Spanish American Children

- De-emphasis on sequencing of events.
- Emphasis on maintaining the flow of conversation among participants over telling a monologic, story-focused narrative (Meltzi, 2000).
- In some Spanish American cultures, narration consists less of telling about punctate past events ("We hit the ball hard") and more of telling about habitual or background activities ("We were hitting the ball around . . .").
- In some Spanish American cultures, narrators mention extended family members frequently to let listeners know about the narrator; such connections between extended family and what, where, and when some experience was happening can sound tangential to non-Hispanic listeners but are the point of narration to some Hispanic speakers.
- Switching from Spanish to English and vice versa.
- Some dysfluencies in English as a result of learning a second language.

—adapted from Silva & McCabe, 1996

Example Narratives from Children with Typical Language Development

Spanish-speaking Americans hail from numerous different countries, each with its own distinct culture. What follows are just a sampling of narratives from diverse Spanish-speaking children. We have a larger sampling from Mexican American children, due to Lynn Bliss.

Example from 7-year-, 5-month-old bilingual boy from El Salvador
(given in English, from our files)

Interviewer: (*Tells brief personal narrative about bee sting*) What about you? Have you ever gotten stung by anything?

Child: All the time in the brown house when I lived here. Got stung, stung, and stung. Because I was, my room was by the porch and all the bees come in and stung me . . . I don't know how they get in, but the do somethin' how to get in . . . I woke up and I saw me all stinged. I was all stinged.

Interviewer: You were all stinged. Then what happened. Tell me more about that.

Child: Then my brother got stinged. He got, he got a little bit on him and me too. But it didn't hurt when he got all pinched . . . I scratched it all the time and it growed because it hurts.

Key points regarding this narrative are:

- Asked to elaborate the story about himself getting stung, this child elects to tell about his brother's contrastive experience instead. There is no resolution about what was or was not done to medicate his stings; he prefers to speak of a similar experience (not necessarily the same time) that happened to his sibling—a tendency we found quite often in children from Caribbean and Central American cultures.
- There are a few signs that English is this child's second language, albeit the one he is most fluent in. For example, he omits a pronoun, common in Spanish, when he gives the high point event: "[I] got stung, stung, and stung."
- Sequencing of events is not emphasized here. Instead the narrator gives us a memorable description of his discovery of his wound: "I woke up and I saw me all stinged." The details and point of this story are to make vivid an experience of the narrator and a contrastive, yet similar, one of his brother.

Example from 6-year-, 4-month-old bilingual boy from El Salvador
(given in Spanish, translated below, from our files)

Interviewer: (*Tells brief personal narrative*) Do you know any cats?

Child: (*Nods yes*) That I was going to grab it and it went running. I was running to catch it. I was almost catching it and, and [it] kept running even faster, but I could not get to [it]. [I] did not get to it.

Key points include:

- This narrative is notable for its reliance upon the past progressive (e.g., "was going") rather than simple past tense, a common practice among Spanish-speaking children. Reliance upon the past progressive means that there is overall less emphasis on a clear sequence of events. In this case, there is no true, formal sequence of past-tense events at all (the definition of narrative, according to Labov, 1972), and yet there is certainly a story here.

- There are several omissions of pronouns, also acceptable in Spanish, since the subject of the sentence is easily inferred.
- This is a narrative about something that did *not* happen—the one that got away.

To give readers a sense of narrative development in children from Mexican American homes, we begin by giving some typical examples. All the children in this chapter come from bilingual homes with Spanish as their first language.

Example Narratives from Spanish-English Bilingual Children with Typical Language Development*

Oral narrative—4-year-old Mexican American boy (from our files)
I got stinged by a je—I got stinged when I was going to the beach with my dad. I got stinged by a jellyfish. And there was a big mark, and know, know what? I was crying a lot. When I got stinged by a jellyfish, I cried. And then, know what? My dad bought me medicine and then I wasn't crying any more. I didn't cry any more.

Key points regarding this narrative are:

- This narrative conforms to what Peterson and McCabe (1983) called "classic" narrative style for European North American children. Typically, European American children engage in such narration at the age of 6 years, so this child is performing well above his age level.
- The narrative contains evaluation ("I cried a lot"), orientation ("when I was going to the beach with my dad"), and action ("I got stinged by a jelly fish"). Note that "stinged" is an overregularization characteristic of typical child language in any culture (Brown, 1973).

Oral narrative—5-year-old Mexican American girl (from our files)
I go to the dentist and I brush my tooth. The dentist say, "Brush you teeth right here and right here and right here and everywhere." And then my mommy went her teeth too. My mommy name Mara and my daddy name José. I got flowers at home. And I got a Barbie bed. And then my mom, my mommy was working hard, but my mom picked me up and then my dad picked me up. Because actually my teacher picked me up at home. And then and then Gianna I go to her house. You wanna hear a song the Mickey Mouse?

The key points about this narrative are:

- This narrative is about going to the dentist on only the most superficial level. The girl's real point is to tell her listener several important facts about her family—the names of her parents, her mom's trip to the dentist, too, some

---

* Unless otherwise noted, narratives were produced in English.

valuable things she has at home, and how hard her mother works. Such an approach is often found in the narratives of children from various Spanish backgrounds (Rodino et al., 1991; Silva & McCabe, 1996). Listeners not from this tradition may misunderstand such departures from action to be tangential, but they are, as in this case, intended to be the main point of the story. Actions are simply a backdrop to the information revealed about the family.

• Nonetheless, note that several events do take place in this narrative (going to the dentist, brushing teeth, getting picked up, etc.).

Oral narrative—6-year-old Mexican American girl (from our files)
My mom took me in [to the hospital] in the car. And then we stop in the hospital and then, and me mom put me in in. And the hospital man and put some shots. And and and then, I scream myself and cry. And then, and then, and then I put a Band-Aid and it's okay. And I put my clothes right in my mouth and then I can't hurt. And and and then, I can, I can . . . And then and then I cough and the sneeze and I am very sick. And then I went to hospital and stay here. And and Tramora he can take me home. And then and then, the hospital check me and me and me stomach. And then he and then he. . . . check it and stuck it and stuck it out—the cough and the sneeze. And then I feel much better and told the hospital I can take the medicine. And then they said yes. And eat some candy.

This bilingual child is still mastering the use of the past tense, among other constructions, in English and occasionally buys time to plan her next sentence by repeating conjunctions (*and, and then*). She meets the standard for oral narration in K–1 (see *Speaking and Listening from Preschool through Third Grade*, discussed in Chapter 2):
Key points include:

• She gives enough setting information to define who was involved (her mother and her and the hospital man). She specifies relevant objects (Band-Aids, candy).
• Evaluation is concentrated in the middle, where the narrator clearly describes expressing her pain by screaming and crying and trying to stuff clothes in her mouth to keep herself from screaming more. She coughs and sneezes and is "very sick."
• Motivation is clearly implied; she tells the hospital she can take the medicine, so they say "yes" and she also gets treated to some candy.
• She resolves the experience: "And then I feel much better."

Oral narrative—8-year-old bilingual Mexican American boy (from our files)
No, [I have not had a snakebite], but my cousin did. In Mexico. It, cause he was playing on the grass and then there was a snake right there—hid inside. He just saw something black like walking around. He didn't know. He just kept on running and then the snake bit him on the leg. They had to take him to a hospital. Then they put him—something I don't remember. And then he came back home and then he couldn't go outside anymore cause he think he might get bitten by the same snake.

That's why he can't go outside anymore. Then they finally let him go outside and when he went outside, he saw the same snake and he saw it. And he saw the same snake! He grab a stick and he hit it with it. He just hit it with the stick. He grab a stick and he hit it with it. He just hit with the stick cause he got mad. But the snake just kept on running and then he grabbed something like a knife and killed it.

Although this child is still in the process of learning English, and therefore does not always form the past tense accurately, he meets the standards for narration in grades 2–3. Specifically:

- The setting information is explicit about who (cousin, snake), what (stick, something like a knife), and where (in Mexico) the events occurred.
- Evaluation is concentrated by several repetitions of key elements at the climax, which is when the boy's cousin saw the snake again ("He saw the same snake and he saw it. And he saw the same snake! He hit it with it. He just hit it with the stick. He grab a stick and he hit it with it. He just hit with the stick cause he got mad").
- He tells us how the experience was resolved: The snake was killed.
- Characters' motivations are explicit (". . . he couldn't go outside anymore cause he think he might get bitten by the same snake. . . . He just hit with the stick cause he got mad").
- Although the child gives no coda, the end of the story is clear.
- This is a narrative that is appropriately long, with enough elaboration to satisfy listeners.
- The actions of sighting the snake and hits are repeated for evaluative reasons. However, there are more than ten different events told in chronological order.
- Ongoing events are described (cousin kept on running at first; later the snake just kept on running).
- The cousin's goal is clearly satisfied: He killed the snake that bit him.

Oral narrative—10-year-old Mexican American boy (from our files)
Adult: Have you ever been in a car accident?

Sam: Um . . . there was a van, a truck, and a car that had crashed and there was a red car that was crushed and the truck uh it had a flat tire that fell and it had some broken window.

Some salient points about this narrative include:

- Although the narrator describes little action per se, the listener understands that events occurred.
- This narrator uses mostly description and evaluation (e.g., red, flat, broken). While this type of narrative, characterized by infrequent actions, has been previously described for Central American and Caribbean children (Rodino et al., 1991), the samples we collected from Mexican American children do not typically show this reduced number of events.

Typical Narrative Development

The Spanish-speaking community in the United States includes diverse cultures and subcultures, originating primarily from Central and South America, Puerto Rico, Cuba, Mexico, Texas, and California. Variations among and within these cultures are evident (Silva & McCabe, 1996). Unfortunately, there is insufficient research to enable us to identify possible distinguishing or common traits among the narratives of all the different cultures of Spanish-speaking children. Professionals need to realize that variations most likely exist among and within different Spanish-speaking communities. In this chapter, we will focus on the narratives produced by children from southeastern Texas, who first learned Spanish at home. Mexican Americans account for 62.6 percent of the Hispanic population as of the 1992 census, by far the largest subset of this population (U.S. Bureau of the Census, 1992).

In the past three years we have collected narrative samples from Spanish-speaking children from Mexican American backgrounds in Texas. We collected samples from children with typical or impaired language development. The children with impaired development had been diagnosed as impaired by bilingual speech-language pathologists after being tested at their schools using language measures that were normed on Spanish speakers [e.g., *The Woodcock Language Proficiency Battery: Spanish Form* (Woodcock, 1981) and the *Expressive One-Word Picture Vocabulary Test* (Gardner, 1983)]. All the children diagnosed as language impaired were receiving remedial language services. Personal narratives were elicited in both English and in Spanish using the Conversational Map Procedure (McCabe & Rollins, 1994). The narratives presented here are those that were elicited in English. We established that narratives were nearly identical in English and Spanish (Bliss, McCabe, & Mahecha, 2000), which is an example of the transfer of language skills that is routinely documented for bilingual children (Cummins, 1991).

The Mexican American children whose narratives appeared at the outset of this chapter learned English informally as a second language. That is, they did not receive formal instruction in English at school, but instead "picked it up" by interacting with family and friends at home. The characteristics of their narratives may be different from those of speakers from different Spanish-speaking cultural backgrounds, even in the United States.

Another consideration is the existence of language mixing that is prevalent among bilingual and/or multilingual speakers' language (Long, 1994). Some bilingual individuals have developed two languages through simultaneous acquisition prior to the age of 3, with some favoring of each language in different contexts (Grosjean, 1982). More common is successive acquisition; children learn one language at home (L1) and a second language (L2) in school and/or with peers after the age of 3 (Owens, 1996). The acquisition of more than one language is a dynamic process in which different languages generally influence each other (Cummins, 1984). The degree of proficiency in each language will change as children mature. A typical pattern has been identified for Spanish-speaking children in the United States who are learning English as their second language. In general, children will perform better in their second language as they progress in school, and this shift in their levels of proficiency will affect their narration as well as their syntax, phonology, and vocabulary (Gutiérrez-Clellen, 1996, Gutiérrez-Clellen et al., 2000).

Features of Bilingual Spanish-English Narratives

Before we examine specific features of narratives spoken by bilingual Spanish-English speakers, it is necessary to discuss the general form of narratives that many bilingual individuals use (Heath, 1986). Vasquéz (1989) described the communication patterns of four Mexican American families. Story retelling, which was the main communication event in the home, was used for entertainment. A variety of other patterns were evident, including the exchange of stories from folklore, family events, and descriptions of past experiences. The role of parents was to maintain conversation, rather than to teach or correct their children's attempts. Food preparation in Mexican American families is frequently used as a time for storytelling (Silva & McCabe, 1996). Spanish Americans value participating in discourse more than relaying specific information or describing a series of events (Melzi, 2000; Silva & McCabe, 1996).

Topic Maintenance

The narratives of some Spanish speakers may include frequent mention and descriptions of family members, as has been found with individuals from Caribbean and South American backgrounds (Rodino et al., 1991). Reference to family members is a means of providing cohesion within the narrative and of specifying time and place (Rodino et al., 1991; Uccelli, 1997) and sometimes evaluation. Individuals who are not from a speaker's culture might think that the topic was not maintained because of the tendency to specify family members in lieu of sequencing events. However, reference to family members is a narrative device used to ground the narrator and listener (Rodino et al., 1991).

Conversation-focus stories may be prevalent in some Spanish-speaking households (Melzi, 1997, 2000). In this conversation-focused style, mothers keep conversations with their children flowing but are not especially concerned with finding out a particular sequence of events that happened in the past.

Puerto Rican Spanish-speaking adults often tell narratives that combine several experiences into one narrative, while English speakers almost never talk about more than one experience at a time (Peréz, 1998; Peterson & McCabe, 1983).

Event Sequencing

We must be cautious not to overgeneralize these data because there are cultural and linguistic variations across Spanish-speaking groups. Some researchers (e.g., Peréz, 1998, for Puerto Rican adults) have found no differences between Spanish and English speakers in the percentage of personal narratives devoted to depicting actions. In other cases, however, speakers may de-emphasize actions and event sequencing, in particular Spanish-speaking children from Central America or the Caribbean (Rodino, Gimbert, Peréz, Craddock-Willis, & McCabe, 1991). The de-emphasis or backgrounding of event sequencing reflects a preference for using a style that emphasizes different narrative features, such as description, location, and evaluation of experiences (Silva & McCabe, 1996).

Another feature of the narratives of some Spanish speakers is the frequent use of the progressive form and present verb tense (Sebastian & Slobin, 1994; Wong Fillmore, 1976). The frequent use of the progressive form and the present tense may be related to commonly used constructions of the Spanish language (Sebastian & Slobin, 1994). Spanish actions that are completed as well as those in progress can be produced as progressive forms (Sebastian & Slobin, 1994). The differences in the formulation of verb tenses in Spanish and the preferences for the present tense and the progressive form may result in the backgrounding of event sequencing in narration by some Spanish speakers (Silva & McCabe, 1996).

Informativeness

Police officer's needs: Do you understand the incident that the speaker is trying to relate?   Spanish narratives contain just as many words—one measure of informativeness—as English narratives (Peréz, 1998). Listeners should be able to understand the incident a speaker is trying to relate. However, bear in mind that when people are acquiring a second language, they may struggle at times with their new vocabulary, and this may compromise the clarity of what they are trying to say. Professionals will want to take pains to ensure that they do not mistake the typical struggles of becoming bilingual for deficiencies.

Teacher's goals: Did the speaker give ample detail or just the bare bones of the incident?   As the examples at the outset of this chapter reveal, Spanish-English bilingual children often elaborate their personal narratives. However, they may elaborate by providing detail about connections between experiences and family and friends rather than going into detail about objects or events.

Chef's ingredients: Are action, orientation, and evaluation present?   All three ingredients should be present in the narratives of even young children, although as we have mentioned, orientation and evaluation may eclipse the actions narrated. Older children include more narrative actions than younger children (Gutiérrez-Clellen & Iglesias, 1992).

Referencing

Gutiérrez-Clellen and Heinrichs-Ramos (1993) studied the referential cohesion of narratives of a film by Puerto Rican Spanish-speaking children aged 4, 6, and 8 years. All the children introduced the main characters of the movie in their stories. The older they were, the more they tended to include references to props and the location of events in their stories. Furthermore, children produced proportionately more appropriate phrases when introducing referents and significantly fewer inappropriate reintroductory and ambiguous phrases. Personal narratives produced in Spanish by Puerto Rican adults contain a significantly greater percentage of reference cohesion than do those produced by English-speaking adults (Peréz, 1998).

Professionals should keep in mind that agents or sentence subjects are often omitted in Spanish, as referential information may be derived from the inflectional endings of verbs (Gutiérrez-Clellen & Heinrichs-Ramos, 1993). This habit of ellipsis is often imported into their second language, English, although those inflections are missing.

Conjunctive Cohesion

As the examples at the outset of this chapter reveal, bilingual children use abundant and varied conjunctions in their personal narratives. This is true regardless of which language they use. Personal narratives contain equivalent amounts of conjunctive cohesion in Spanish and English (Peréz, 1998).

Gutiérrez-Clellen and Iglesias (1992) found that most Puerto Rican Spanish-speaking children aged 4, 6, and 8 years produced some causal connections in their narratives. With increasing age, causal chains became more complex; children began to interconnect up to six clauses in causal sequences.

Fluency

Peréz (1998) found that English-speaking monolingual adults take much longer to start a narrative than do Puerto Rican Spanish speakers, yet the Spanish narratives contained a significantly greater percentage of false starts and corrections and within-narrative pauses and silences. Delays in responding to a conversational partner are considered rude in Spanish but not English. Thus, in Spanish, speakers do less planning up front and more during the process of narration, whereas in English there is more preplanning of the discourse since delays in response do not have the same connotation. This means that professionals need to look at the overall pattern of dysfluencies—their location in discourse as well as their presence—when working with Spanish-English bilingual individuals.

Dysfluencies may also be a characteristic of second-language learning and not reflective of a disorder (Gutiérrez-Clellen, 1996), as in the following narrative that we collected:

> ### Narrative—6-year-old Spanish-English bilingual boy
> **Adult:**　Have you ever been to the hospital?
>
> **Child:**　I was um . . . There was um a doctor because . . . there was some, uh, somebody in trouble. They were in trouble.
>
> **Adult:**　They were in trouble?
>
> **Child:**　Somebody.

Adult: Somebody? Tell me more.

Child: Um . . . Danielle, she go to hospital . . . and there was um . . . there and and the hospital in trouble . . . um . . . um . . . the man . . . and there was some . . . The hospital because . . . There was um . . . this hospital . . . and the and the girl was sleepy and the bed with his dad.

This child's narrative is characterized by many pauses, fillers, word and phrasal repetitions, and abandoned utterances. These dysfluencies, which are evident to a lesser degree in the narratives of children with typical language development, make his narrative difficult to understand, but are not ipso facto a sign of pathology because interviews with his parents and teachers *consistently revealed that the child was fluent in his first language, Spanish.* His dysfluencies in English were indicative of difficulty accessing appropriate English words.

Example Narratives from Spanish-English Bilingual Children with Impaired Language Development

Minimal narration will most commonly be evident from children with language impairments, characterized by a reduced number of utterances or the inability to produce a narrative (Miranda, McCabe, & Bliss, 1998). In the following sample, a child with a language impairment can barely produce a narrative.

Example from 9-year-old girl with specific language impairment (SLI)
Adult: Have you ever spilled anything?

Child: I spilled water.

Adult: What happened?

Child: I cleaned it up.

Adult: Tell me more.

Child: That's all.

Adult: Anything else?

Child: No.

Topic Maintenance: Appropriate. The two sentences pertain to a single incident.

Event Sequencing: Appropriate. She presents two events in the order in which they occurred.

Informativeness: Inappropriate. While we understand this slim narrative, informativeness is the area of this child's greatest difficulty. She provides us with no elaboration, no details that would distinguish this experience as her own. She presents two events, but no description or evaluation. That is, we don't know whether the water was hot or cold, where she spilled it, what she spilled it out of, who might or might not have seen her, nor how she felt about spilling it.

Referencing: Appropriate, if minimal. She specifies herself with a pronoun and water by that name first, followed appropriately by pronominal reference to it.

Conjunctive Cohesion: Inappropriate. She does not use any conjunctions.

Fluency: Appropriate. She is fluent in her brief narrative.

This child is only able to provide two narrative statements. We would expect a longer and more descriptive recount from a 9-year-old child.

Intervention Goals.   This child's narrative is similar in style to the narratives produced by many children with SLI. She needs to produce longer and more informative narratives. Elaboration and critical narrative ingredients need to be modeled and elicited.

Many of the children with language impairments in our sample produced brief narratives. However, there was variability among this group of children. For example, contrast this child's narrative with the following one from another child who was also diagnosed as language impaired.

> *Example from 10-year-old girl with specific language impairment (from our files)*
> **Adult:** Have you ever spilled anything?
>
> **Child:** (1) OK, first I was hummm, first I got a uh I got a bowl of oh mmm and I got to put it on the table with some milk and some cereal and then I was eating. (2) Then my brother was drop it (3) and my mom didn't hit me. (4) She just get mad at me, (5) fall down 'cause bigger, bigger, bigger than my brother. (6) I mean so so you have to clean. (7) Today my sister, she she was . . . (8) We buy something at McDonalds and some drinks, some drinks for our to clean ourselves. (9) We had to clean it. (10) That's it. What she said, "You have to go to bed right now." (11) In the morning, my brother, he was drinking some orange (12) so get uh some coke. (13) It was all filled up, (14) got the mop and clean it and and tired of doing everything, (15) so she send us to sleep, (16) drink our bottle then we get water (17) and then we time out in the wall and (18) "Don't come out in thirty minutes." (19) That's what she said. (20) We all drop some coke that all my sister mmm (21) she she she got she got water and (22) she was trying to bring it in the room (23) and when she put it on top of the thing (24) she she she was going to the restroom. (25) Then my little brother, he climbed up at the chair and dropped it on the rug (26) and my mom got mad of him, José, (27) because because she put it on top of the thing (28) and she shouldn't have put it in the kitchen (29) so she she got put time out. (30) She put Javi, my brother, down, so he could go to sleep.

Even though this narrative is difficult for some professionals to follow, it exhibits many strengths, as the child was able to relate a lively and generally meaningful narrative with a variety of events and people.

Topic Maintenance: Appropriate. English-speaking monolingual professionals may be puzzled because the narrative contains many spilling episodes. However, this attribute reveals that the child is using a conversational focused narrative structure. This should not be considered to be an impairment. All her comments pertain to spilling and the consequences of spilling.

Event Sequencing: Appropriate. The child tells many events in sequence throughout the narrative (e.g., 21–29).

Informativeness: Variable. The most serious difficulty with this narrative is that the speaker omits many events. For example, in 8 and between 13 and 14 she omits the actual spill. The listener must do considerable work to understand the basic facts of most of the incidents she describes.

In terms of elaboration, she provides some detail for each of the incidents, although more details would make the account more engaging. This is not as serious an omission as the previous one.

This narrative is rich with actions. There is some evaluation ("my mom got mad of him, José"; note that prepositions in second languages (e.g., *of*) are often easily confused—not a sign of impairment). There is also some description ("It was all filled up"). However, the narrator might well be encouraged to provide more evaluation and description, as well as the requisite events mentioned earlier.

Referencing: Variable. The child does not always use agents (e.g., 5, 14, and the beginning section of 16), which is a feature of Spanish, as we noted previously; she may transfer this Spanish-speaking syntactic rule into her English usage, so that is not a problem per se. She also often introduces participants specifically ("my brother" in 2, "my mom" in 3) and then uses pronouns appropriately. ("She just get mad at me" in 4). Again, note that tense is a struggle for second language learners and is not a sign of impairment. However, the agent or agents in 14 are very unclear, but probably it is the mother, not the brother, who was the last referent specified.

Conjunctive Cohesion: Appropriate. The narrator uses many and varied conjunctions: *so* (12, 15, 30), *and then* (17), *then* (2, 25), *and* (3, 26), and *because* (27).

Fluency: Needs further study. The narrative contains false starts at the outset, abandoned utterances (20), and repetitions (21). However, in view of the cautions we have made about dysfluencies due to typical second language acquisition issues, as well as in Spanish narration generally, the assessment of this dimension must remain open. Consultation with the child's parents and/or other familiar adults could provide professionals with information about whether she ordinarily engages in typical or atypical dysfluency.

Intervention Goals.   The speaker needs to produce a clearer narrative. This child needs to become more sensitive to the discourse needs of the listener. Through contingent queries and modeling, the child can learn to give sufficient information for the listener to fully understand her narration.

Example from 10-year-, 3-month-old boy with mental retardation (from our files)
Adult: I saw an awful car accident. Have you ever seen a car accident?

Child: Doesn't look very well. But there was a guy inside of a car. So look, there, there was this other car right here. This other car came, car up and tried, the the guy tried to stop. He couldn't stop because the brake, his brake, the front, the brake over here—the one you try to stop with. He put the thing but it wouldn't stop, so it hit the car and then the ambulance came and got the guy out of the car. They took him and then they put, they put him in that thing. That thing, that thing where they put you in. Where you hurt at. So then they took him to the room and left him there. So then next week he got out, and he was okay. And so that's how he didn't get hurt for another week. He didn't drive the car for another week cause his hand was broke right here (points to where hand was broken). His leg was broke. That's why he wasn't hurt that much. This side was okay, this leg. But, um, next week the officer told him not to drive the car for two weeks. So, he didn't drive the car for two weeks. Yesterday his wife had to take him. His kids stayed home. So then his wife drove the car. His wife, she got into an accident. She, she took him to work. Then she, she tried to get to work, but there was another guy in the parking lot. And she was trapped. She couldn't, she couldn't she couldn't move the car back or front because she was trapped. All the other cars, the other cars were parked. She was stuck there forever.

Adult: Oh. Anything else?

Child: Well there's one thing. Maybe if she doesn't get hurt again, she can't drive the car. If she can drive the car she won't be hurt. If she can drive the car for a week.

Topic Maintenance: Appropriate. This narrative is a recapitulation of two related accidents.

Event Sequencing: Appropriate. The narrator presents numerous sequences of events in plausible order (e.g., "it hit the car and then the ambulance came and got the guy out of the car . . .").

Informativeness: Variable. Not enough information or contradictory information make this narrative difficult to understand (e.g., "Maybe if she doesn't get hurt again, she can't drive the car. If she can drive the car, she won't be hurt"). The narrator's elaboration is sufficient, but could be more extensive. All three ingredients are present: evaluation (e.g., "Doesn't look very well"), description (e.g., "there was this other car right here"), and action (e.g., "the guy tried to stop").

Referencing: Variable. The narrator introduces some participants with adequate specificity (e.g., "a guy inside a car," "his wife," "his kids"). However, there is some problematic referencing ("He put *the thing*, but *it* wouldn't stop, so *it* hit the car"). This could be due to word-finding problems of second-language acquisition or disorder. Ellipsis of "the accident" at the outset of the narrative is acceptable, perhaps a carryover from Spanish subject ellipsis.

Conjunctive Cohesion: Appropriate. The narrator uses *but, and then, and so, so then,* and *because* accurately and often.

Fluency: Appropriate. In a few places, the narrator repeats part of a phrase several times ("that thing, that thing, that thing where they put you in" and "She couldn't, she couldn't, she couldn't"). In view of the information presented earlier about the occurrence of dysfluencies in typical Spanish narration, professionals would be well advised to see this as acceptable.

Intervention Goals.   This child needs to provide more accurate, clear information to the listener. The child also needs to provide appropriate references to the people that he mentions in his narratives.

> *Example from 12-year-, 9-month-old bilingual Mexican American girl with traumatic brain injury (from our files)*
>
> **Adult:**   . . . Have you ever gotten in a fight with someone?
>
> **Child:**   Oh . . . yeah . . . My brother . . . Um, My cousin, he, he's Manuel. He fights with me all the time. He picks on me too. And the other time I was, I was asleep. And, and, then, he, he went to go get a flower. And then he, he put it on my nose. Now (sniffs). And, and it got stuck in my, in my nose. And then I woke up. Then I go, I go, I touch my nose if I got anything. 'Cause I was feeling something. And then, and then I go and I took it out. And then I say. And I got up and Manuel was there. And I went and I went over there and hit him, hit him. And he hits me back. But I hit him real hard, like that (gestures) in the stomach. And he got mad. And that's it.

Topic Maintenance: Appropriate. The narrative recounts a fight straightforwardly.

Event Sequencing: Appropriate. (e.g., "He went to go get a flower, and then he, he put it on my nose . . .").

Informativeness: Variable. Have we enough information to make sense of the experience? Not without doing more work than we should have to. That is, there are some odd partial omissions (e.g., "I touch my nose *to see* if I got anything *up it*," where italicized words reflect inferences on our part that would be necessary to comprehend the sentence, and the unfinished sentence, "And then I say"). Elaboration is adequate. All three narrative ingredients are present: evaluation ("And he got mad"), description ("I was asleep"), and action ("He put it on my nose"; note that the preposition *on* is not accurate due to second-language acquisition issues.

Referencing: Appropriate. Manuel is first specified by name, followed by pronominal reference.

Conjunctive Cohesion: Appropriate. The narrator uses *and* and *and then* frequently, *because* and *but* accurately.

Fluency: Inappropriate because the child is also very dysfluent in Spanish, which was ascertained from interviews with parents and teachers. Virtually every sentence contains repetition of some of its words ("And, and . . . he, he . . . he, he . . . in my, in my . . . I go, I go, and then and then, I went and I went . . . hit him, hit him"). We cannot dismiss this level of repetition, clearly not for evaluative purposes, as due to second-language acquisition or to Spanish discourse style because it is so extensive.

Intervention Goals. The child needs to provide more information in her narrative. Fluency can be targeted as a secondary goal.

Assessment Considerations

Even though children may speak predominately English at home, some common features of Spanish narration may be present in their personal narratives. We have seen this Spanish influence in the narratives produced by Spanish-speaking bilingual children. For example, some of their narratives are characterized by the inclusion of family members, broadly defined topic maintenance, and referencing grounded by the mention of family members. This pattern shows a Spanish influence on narration even though the language used is English. Cultural preferences for discourse patterns may carry over to other languages spoken.

Children may be unaware of what is expected in school concerning the form of narratives. Their narrative traditions and models in the home must be accepted as legitimate forms of sense making (Rosen, 1985). Children should be encouraged to tell myths and legends, such as "La Llorona," and describe family relationships and experiences.

A questionnaire is useful to determine the language experiences and exposure of a bilingual child (see Chapter 7). Professionals need to know the types of discourse that are used in the child's home. In addition, the amount of exposure to each of the child's languages should be determined.

When conducting assessment of children from some Spanish backgrounds, using impersonal prompts may be particularly ill-advised. Professionals may come across as cold unless they make some mention of genuine personal experiences. We are not suggesting that professionals tell anything that would make them uncomfortable. But mention of some personal relationships (e.g., "After I had lunch with my sister, . . .") may serve as a useful connection to children being interviewed.

Topic Maintenance

Some Spanish children include family members to identify events and people in their narratives. This discourse style may appear to reflect reduced topic maintenance, as tangential themes have been introduced. Adults need to accept variations in topic maintenance with Spanish speakers, especially when family members are included (Silva & McCabe, 1996). An example of the emphasis on family was revealed in a transcript in which a mother is talking to her 3-year-old child in Spanish. The mother frequently asked the child questions about family members, including siblings, her parents, grandparents, and cousins instead of the events that are so often the focus of conversations in European North American families.

Event Sequencing

Reduced action and sequencing should not be considered signs of impaired narration. Some Spanish speakers produce narratives similar to the one about the "red car that was crushed" at the outset of this chapter. He has typical language development and has not chosen to use actions to describe an event. In the samples that we have collected in Texas from children with typical or impaired development, however, the majority included actions. Professionals need to assess all dimensions of narration to determine if a deficit exits.

Informativeness

The narratives of Spanish speakers are expected to be informative and elaborated. There should be a richness of orientation and evaluation. Impaired narration results in habitually short narratives. The aforementioned example of the child who talked about spilling water is an extreme example of lack of informativeness. Children with mild delays, in our data collection project, used all the narrative ingredients (e.g., actions, descriptions, evaluations); children with delay did use significantly fewer actions than their peers with typical language development but did not differ in the production of description or evaluation (Bliss, McCabe, & Mahecha, 2000). Omission of redundant or predictable subjects or agents may be a transference from Spanish and not a reflection of an impairment.

Referencing

Referents that are understood in a context, especially subjects, may be deleted by some Spanish speakers because redundant forms can be omitted in Spanish (Sebastian & Slobin, 1994). General vocabulary use or misuse of referents might indicate a second language learning limitation and not language impairment. Bilingual children may be able to express some ideas more clearly in Spanish than in English.

Bilingual speakers also code-switch from one language into another language. It is often difficult to differentiate between word-finding problems and lack of proficiency in English. Only bilingual clinicians, knowledgeable of both bilingual acquisition processes and language impairments, can make judgments regarding the existence of a pathology. Eliciting and analyzing a language sample in the child's native language and asking a caregiver about the adequacy of the child's lexical and referencing usage in the native language is critical.

Conjunctive Cohesion

Spanish speakers use conjunctions in their narratives. If speakers do not use conjunctions, their narratives are most likely deficient in this dimension. In this chapter the children with language impairments used conjunctions (except for the child who talked of spilling water above). Signs of impairment might be absent, limited, or erroneous use of conjunctions. However, errors may also signal a second-language learning delay and not an impairment. For this reason, a bilingual speech-language pathologist is needed to distinguish limited English proficiency and language impairment.

Fluency

Pauses and hesitations may be evident because a speaker is trying to formulate a narrative in a second language and needs time to find appropriate wording. These pauses may reflect learning a second language and not language impairment. A latency in responding to a question may reflect a child's lack of knowledge about the question or topic or a need to plan discourse. A bilingual informant is critical when assessing a child who speaks more than one language.

Intervention Considerations

It is not the scope of this book to discuss whether intervention should be carried out in the child's first or second language. Numerous papers have been written on this subject (e.g., Brice, 1994; Gutiérrez-Clellen, 1999; Kayser, 1995 a, b). In this section, we will focus briefly on the narrative aspects of intervention that need to be considered when working with Spanish bilingual children.

Family vignettes may be a starting point in intervention if this type of narration is used in the home. A child could be asked to describe family activities, such as preparing food or going to a festival. Inclusion of stories with family members improves verbal performance (Ruíz, 1989). Conversation-focused stories, common to many Spanish-speaking cultures, should also be included (Melzi, 1997; Peréz, 1998). Such stories involve a shifting of focus from one event to another one that happened in the past. An adult maintains a conversation with a child rather than probing for specific information about a particular past experience (Melzi, 1997). A child is not typically encouraged or asked to recount details of a personal experience (Silva & McCabe, 1996). Adults can use conversation stories with children with language impairments by including stories about family members, adventures, aspirations, public figures, and myths. Clinicians can ask parents to tell them the stories that are frequently told at home so that the child can practice them (Silva & McCabe, 1996).

Two-event narratives should be elicited from children who cannot produce them. Later, more elaborate narratives also need to receive focus. Inclusion of actions, sequencing of events, evaluation, and orientation should be highlighted for some children. Children should be told that there are different ways to tell stories, that a different form of narrative may be expected in the school than is used at home. The school form includes many actions that are part of a single experience and are presented chronologically. Children can tell stories that are more like the ones they use at home and then retell them with the structure that is expected in the classroom.

Published stories that are based in a child's culture are also an important resource. Examples are *My Aunt Ottila's Spirits* (Garcia, 1987), *Pablo Remembers: The Fiesta of the Day of the Dead* (Ancona, 1993), *Family Pictures: Cuadores de familia* (Garza, 1990), and *Voices of the Field* (Atkin, 1993). These books can serve as models for children who speak Spanish.

In short, the stories told by Spanish-speaking children are vibrant and rich with meaning. Professionals need bilingual speech-language pathologists to carry out valid assessment of children who speak more than one language. Children's narrative styles may differ and children may be unfamiliar with the genres expected in schools. Clinicians need to preserve the discourse styles found in children's homes and elicit other styles that are expected in schools.

6

Asian American Children

with Masahiko Minami

Expected Features of Narration: Asian American Children

- A preference for conciseness.
- Frequent combination of several experiences into one story.
- A valuing of implication rather than explication.
- Omission of pronouns, which listeners are expected to infer.

—Minami & McCabe, 1991

Example Narratives from Children with Typical Language Development

There are many different Asian cultures represented in the United States, and Asian immigrants are one of our fastest-growing populations (*New York Times*, April 28, 1993). As with any set of cultures, especially those with individual traditions dating to ancient times, Asian cultures bear both some resemblances to and some differences from each other, which we will highlight in the following examples. Note that due to the work of Masahiko Minami, we have a more complete picture of developing narration in Japanese children than we do in children from other Asian cultures.

Perhaps the aspect of narration in many Asian cultures that poses the greatest challenge to Westerners is the preference for implication. Habitual omission of pronouns, which we will see much of in the examples that follow, may well strike European North American listeners as impaired narration. In fact, children who practice such omission have been very well socialized by their families into the style of narration preferred by Eastern cultures, where listeners are expected to be more active than in Western ones. Consider the following:

> ***Example from 7-year-old Chinese boy living in the United States***
> ***(collected, transcribed, translated, and analyzed by Chien-Ju Chang, 1994;***
> ***words in parentheses were not spoken by the child)***
> That is . . . I was originally very afraid. Then, (I had a) checkup. The dentist filled up my tooth. After filling up, I did not feel painful. But I came the second time. I felt painful here. Then the dentist said that (one tooth) must be pulled out. So he pulled it out. I was afraid. Then he used drugs . . . Then I was very pained. Pain was gone—he asked me. Then he asked me to rinse the mouth. After rinsing, he pulled it out again. Finally, once more. This time (he) put the tooth in my mouth. Gold Tooth. This one (shows interviewer).

Some key points about this narrative include:

- This narrator, like Japanese narrators, as we will see, uses an elliptical style in which pronouns and nouns are often omitted (see information in parentheses denoting such omissions) because listeners can easily infer such information.
- Several experiences (here with the dentist) are combined here, as will also prove true with Japanese narration.
- About a third of the Chinese children interviewed by Chang (1994) ended their narratives at the climactic moment, just as this child did. The high point is clearly the gold tooth he received.

> ***Example from a 7-year-old Korean boy (from our files)***
> A nurse came. With a cotton ball she rubbed. Then I came home. After she rubbed it with a cotton ball, she gave me a present. I got a bandage and I got presents.

Key points include:

- As is the case with the Chinese child and the Japanese children who follow, this Korean boy displays reticence in narration. He gives us the important facts, but does not go into detail.
- As with Japanese children (Minami, 1996), this Korean child sticks primarily to the events of the incident. There is little orientation or evaluation mentioned.

> ***Example from 4-year-old Japanese girl (collected, transcribed, and translated by***
> ***Masahiko Minami; note that ellipsis—the strategic omission of certain easily***
> ***inferable parts of speech—is typical practice in Japanese. Here ellipsis is noted by***
> ***including English items in parentheses.)***
> "(I) bled. (I) had (it) cleaned. That was good. (I) was all right."

Reflective of Japanese cultural values for counting on listeners to infer information rather than requiring narrators to explicitly state more than is necessary, this child gives a succinct recount of an injury experience (Minami & McCabe,

1991). Note that this style would be evident even if this child were speaking English, her other language. Apart from her omission of orientation information she probably assumes her listener already knows (another type of ellipsis), she meets standards for oral narration in preschool.

Specifically, key points about her narrative are that it:

- Provides evaluation: "That was good. (I) was all right."
- Includes two events: "bled. Had cleaned."
- Tells an experience that she did not share with her listener.

Example from 6-year-old Japanese girl (from files of Masahiko Minami)
(1) "When (I) was 3 years old, you know. (2) When (I) was small. (3) Um, when (I) went to a restaurant. (4) fell on the stairs (5) and hit my forehead. (6) And a hospital. (7) Um, a man at the restaurant, (8) who was a nice man, (9) who was a nice man, (10) carried me to the hospital. (11) And at the hospital, you know, (12) had stitches on my head, um, on my forehead."

This child meets many of the standards for first-grade oral narration. Key points here include:

- She gives enough orientation for us to know who was involved (she and the man at the restaurant) and mentions relevant objects (stairs). The first utterances (1–3) orient us as to when the event occurred.
- She concentrates evaluation by repeating her statement about the "man at the restaurant who was a nice man."
- The motivation of the man at the restaurant is clearly implied: He carried her to the hospital for treatment of her forehead.
- There are five events in sequence here: "went, fell, hit, man carried her, had stitches." This child gives us the sense she could easily have supplied another had it seemed relevant.
- She goes beyond the emotional climax to comment on how her injury was resolved: She had stitches on her forehead.

Example from 8-year-old Japanese girl (from files of Masahiko Minami)
(1) When (I was) in kindergarten, (2) (I) got (my) leg caught in a bicycle. (3) (I) got a cut here, here and. (4) wore a cast for about a month. (5) Took a rest for about a week, and (6) Went back again. (7) had a cut here. (8) Fell off an iron bar. (9) Yeah, (I) had two mouths.

Because Japanese narratives are often a collection of similar experiences (Minami & McCabe, 1991), rather than a detailed series of events that comprise one experience, build to a climax, and resolve it (as do so many African American and European North American narratives), this child's narrative may puzzle those unfamiliar with this form of storytelling. Giving a *sequence* of actions is not very important to many Japanese children; this is a case where cultural values need to take precedence over standards that are appropriate for most other groups. This is a unified, coherent story told in the Japanese manner, translated into English (by Masahiko Minami). In a succinct way, this child meets relevant standards for oral narration. Specifically:

- She includes setting information about when the event took place (she was in kindergarten at the time) and relevant objects (e.g., bicycle, cast, iron bar).
- Setting information is presented first.
- Evaluation is concentrated in the memorable metaphor at the end, in which she compares wounds metaphorically to mouths.
- Her narrative is lengthier and more elaborate than younger children's because she has elaborated by giving us two different injuries in one story.
- One series of five actions ("got leg caught, got a cut, wore a cast, took a rest, went back again) is followed by a couple of actions that concerned a different injury ("had a cut, fell off an iron bar").
- Japanese children are taught to expect listeners to fill in information for them (see Minami & McCabe, 1991). We could imagine the background context of riding her bicycle in one case and children playing at a playground in the other. Not one of us really needs to be told that her parents were motivated to take her to a hospital to get treatment for her bicycle injury.

Typical Narrative Development

Topic Maintenance

The most striking culturally distinct aspect of narration in Japanese culture is a preference for combining two or three similar incidents into a single story. Whereas we have seen such combinations as a valid cultural option in African American and Spanish American narration, such combinations are a stated preference among Japanese adults (Minami & McCabe, 1991) and are judged more interesting than narratives of single incidents.

Event Sequencing

Japanese preschool children tend to tell their stories in a sequential style (Minami, 1996), a tendency that extends to adulthood. Japanese adults, by contrast, emphasize nonsequential evaluation and orientation (Minami, 1996).

Informativeness

Police officer's needs: Do you understand the incident the speaker is trying to relate?   Because in Japan (among other Asian cultures), listeners are expected to make considerable effort to understand speakers (Minami & McCabe, 1991), professionals who are not from Asian backgrounds may have difficulty assessing this aspect correctly. From an early age, Japanese children are inducted into the practice of *omoiyari*, or empathy. Adults expect them to put themselves in someone else's position in order to understand others' wants and silently elaborate on what they are told (Azuma, 1986; Clancy, 1986; Doi, 1973; Lebra, 1986; Shigaki, 1987). The flip side of this is that as speakers, Japanese children are frequently interrupted by their mothers after a very short turn at narration (Minami & McCabe, 1995) so that they will not become garrulous, which is seen as insulting to listeners and a sign of stupidity. The bare facts of a Japanese narrative, in other words, are likely less numerous than those of European Americans, African Americans, or Spanish-speaking Americans.

Teacher's goals: Did the speaker give ample detail or just the bare bones of the incident?   When asked to elaborate more on the story of a particular incident, a Japanese child is likely to do so *not* by giving the kinds of details they expect their listeners to furnish, but rather to add accounts of similar incidents. Again, this practice could be misunderstood as changing the subject, particularly by European North Americans, who tell one incident per narrative virtually all the time.

Furthermore, professionals attuned to Western values for lengthy stories do not seem to appreciate the succinctness many Asian children have been taught to practice and value. For example, when some European North American teachers were shown translations of narratives such as those at the outset of this chapter, they expressed concern about the children's competence. One teacher said (Minami, 1990; Minami & McCabe, 1996, p. 77), "These children need help. They need more encouragement. They should be in a different type of program, not only because they themselves need to learn communicative skills, but also because if children who are more advanced are put in the same program, they would get bored."

Rather than mistaking cultural differences in preferences for elaboration as deficits, professionals might instead begin to appreciate them. Working with children from cultures not your own is a lot like sanding wood: Sanding a good piece of wood against the grain results in ugliness, while sanding *with* the grain is the stuff of beautiful craftsmanship. Succinctness has many uses in everything from business to poetry, and helping children already well prepared in this regard to advance their ability to compress considerable information into relatively few words is a valuable goal.

Chef's ingredients: Does the narrative contain events, orientation, and evaluation?   All three key ingredients of narrative are to be found in the narratives of Asian children, such as those at the outset of this chapter, from a very young age (Minami & McCabe, 1991). However, compared to 4-year-olds, 5-year-old Japanese children produce proportionately more evaluation in their narratives—approximately adult levels for this ingredient (Minami, 1996). Young Japanese children focus relatively more on actions than they do either orientation or evaluation, whereas Japanese adults devote most of their narration to orientation and, especially, evaluation (Minami, 1996).

Referencing

In Japanese culture, proverbs such as "Still waters run deep" and "A talkative man is embarrassing" distill a cultural preference for being circumspect, for counting on your listeners to do more work following your train of thought than listeners are expected to do in Western contexts. Consequently, omission of pronouns is common among individuals of all socioeconomic strata (Clancy, 1986; Hinds, 1984; Minami & McCabe, 1991).

Conjunctive Cohesion

The Japanese language has many conjunctions, and many are to be found in Japanese narration (Minami, personal communication). As we have repeatedly emphasized, aspects of language in general and discourse in particular often transfer from one language to another. Asian children combine their sentences in English discourse using a variety of conjunctions.

Fluency

Japanese speakers with typical language are expected to be fluent in their native language. Asian speakers learning English as a second language in America, however, may experience the same disruptions of fluency as Spanish immigrants. That is, when speaking in a second language, there may be many hesitations and/or false starts due to problems finding words or forming syntactic constructions in the second language. Consider the following narrative from a recent Vietnamese immigrant child.

> *Example from a 7-year-old Vietnamese boy (enrolled in an English as a Second Language classroom for two years; example from our files)*
> **Adult:** Two weeks ago, I had to go to the hospital. I had some x rays taken. It took a long time. It was scary. Have you ever been to the hospital?
>
> **Child:** I . . . um . . . sometimes.
>
> **Adult:** Tell me about it.
>
> **Child:** Um . . . He was scared because he thought it would, the doctor would give him a shot. And he was, the doctor didn't give him any shots. His mom was, his mom was a little bit happy because he did a little bit good. And the doctor just wanted to see his bones, what happened to him, and it took a very long time because . . . he had to do something with it. He had to do something with it. And . . . it took a very long time . . . until . . . morning . . . and . . . the doctor gave him a good pat on his shoulder.
>
> **Adult:** The doctor gave him a good pat on his shoulder?
>
> **Child:** (*Nods yes*) Um . . . and they went home. And some, his mom say to his dada that he did really good on the doctor's office.
>
> **Adult:** Tell me more.

Child: And. . . . he . . . he cry a lot in the hospital office . . . and he . . . he was practicing no be scare at the doctor.

Adult: What else happened?

Child: Um . . . he, they had to slept in the hospital and until morning. . . . The doctor did a little bit more on him and then . . . then left . . . and . . . the doctor gave him some pain (medication).

While this narrative includes several positive accomplishments, like those at the outset of this chapter, we include it here because it contains a number of linguistic dysfluencies—revisions, delays before responding, use of nonspecific vocabulary (who is "he" anyway?), repetitions ("He had to do something with it")—the kind of behaviors that some have said can differentiate a child with language disorder from a student who is learning English as a second language (Damico, 1985; Damico, Oller, & Storey, 1983). However, Gutiérrez-Clellan (1996) argued that there is evidence that children who appear to use inappropriate communicative behavior based on school culture expectations may be demonstrating characteristics typical of second-language learners (e.g., revisions, dysfluencies, delayed responses) and/ or previously learned communication styles, *not* disorders. Hence, while the preceding discourse is clearly dysfluent, professionals would be well advised to seek more information before deciding that the child is impaired on this basis. In fact, the child's mother was consulted in this case. She reported that her son was not dysfluent in Vietnamese, the language spoken at home.

Characteristics of Impaired Narrative Discourse

While we regret that we do not have specific examples of narration for Asian or Asian American individuals with impairment, we do have some general observations. Bilingual speech language pathologists have asked Japanese children who are struggling with language acquisition questions about past experiences ("What did you do yesterday?"). They have also shown such children sequential pictures and asked them to give explanations. Responding to questions such as "What did you do yesterday?" preschool children with developmental delay do not understand the meaning of "yesterday" and simply talk about their experiences in the past. In other words, they sometimes mix "yesterday" with "last month" (i.e., they use the expression "yesterday" when they talk about the experience that they had a month ago). This usage relates to their understanding about the flow of time (or temporal sequence), and it rarely happens that they explain their experiences in orderly sequence. The extent to which they can narrate about their past experience depends on the degree of each individual child's developmental delay, but the general tendency is that they only talk about what were particularly impressive experiences and they do that piecemeal. Eliciting narratives is often difficult.

With regard to making up a story in response to sequential pictures, children tend to describe each individual picture without referring to the sequence per se; however, this tendency has been documented for young children with typical language from a variety of other cultures (Berman & Slobin, 1994). Some children can use conjunctions. The fact that children can use conjunctions does not necessarily mean that they can explain what happened to them in a logical manner. Thus, it is sometimes questionable that they fully grasp the meaning or function of the conjunction they use.

Assessment Considerations

General Guidelines

When assessing children from Asian communities, we must remember that Asian communities are not homogenous. Descriptions of different Asian communities are presented by Cheng (1991). Differences in languages as well as communicative and cultural values and expectations occur among the varieties of regions in Asia and in the United States. Unfortunately, research is lacking regarding differences among and within Asian communities.

There is not enough information regarding the narratives from Asian individuals who are language impaired. Clinicians need to inquire about the nature of narrative interaction and communicative values in a speaker's home. Specifically, is conciseness taught and valued? If so, children may not be familiar with an elaborated narrative style. They should not be penalized for producing an unelaborated style, one with which they are unfamiliar.

As we have said, we do not have the basis to make systematic comparisons between typical and impaired narrative discourse in Asian languages. To compound this problem, there are not enough bilingual professionals who speak the different languages found in Asian American communities. We need to rely on members of an individual's community to assist us in interpreting and judging narrative abilities.

In this section, assessment guidelines will be presented based on the narratives that we know the most about, those from Japanese-speaking individuals. The narratives have been elicited from speakers with typical language development. We will make conjectures about the nature of disordered Japanese narration. Generalizations to other Asian languages should only be made with consultation from native speakers of a specific language.

Topic Maintenance

Typical narration in Japanese is generally characterized by a series of related experiences rather than a description of one experience (Minami & McCabe, 1996). If a child describes a series of experiences rather than one event, this discourse style should not be considered as impaired. This style is different from the style expected in European North American culture, but should be accepted as part of a speaker's cultural communicative style.

Impaired topic maintenance would be characterized by abrupt changes in topic with descriptions of unrelated events. If a listener from the child's community cannot understand the links between events or if the narrator cannot explain the links that were described, impaired topic maintenance would be suspected.

Event Sequencing

Japanese children are expected to sequence events in the narratives that they use. If there is a violation of the ordering of actions, impairment in this dimension is likely.

Informativeness

Informativeness varies in the narratives of Japanese speakers. Speakers with typical language development will purposefully leave out information that can easily be inferred by sympathetic listeners. The resultant narrative is not expected to be informative in the sense valued by the European North American culture. Again, a Japanese or Japanese American listener is expected to infer many details in a narrative. Western teachers' emphasis on elaboration may have to be reconsidered with such students.

Japanese narratives contain all three ingredients required for narration—description, action, and evaluation. The techniques of evaluating narrative may be more circumscribed than listeners are accustomed to in the Western tradition.

Impaired informativeness is difficult to determine and would best be identified by members of a speaker's community. However, this notion is more complicated than it might seem for bilingual individuals. For example, verbosity, which is not usually valued in Asian communication, may occur and may not be a sign of impairment. Instead, a talkative speaker with an Asian background may have learned the expectations of the European North American community.

Referencing

Referencing by children with typical language development may be characterized by the absence of identifying information because a speaker is trying to be concise. In the narratives presented in this chapter, there were many examples of the acceptable absence of subjects and some objects.

Impaired referencing would be characterized by the absence of nonredundant referents and/or the inappropriate use of referents (e.g., *he* for *she*). If a knowledgeable listener were not able to retrieve the meaning of an absent referent, it might signal an inability of the narrator to know when referents should be included and when they should be omitted. The speaker might not have appropriate presuppositional skills. The appropriateness of the absence of referents should be judged by a member of the speaker's community.

Conjunctive Cohesion

Conjunctions should be present in the narratives of Japanese speakers with typical language development to emphasize temporal or semantic ordering of events.

Fluency

Fluent production is expected in the narratives of speakers with typical language development. Dysfluencies may not signal an impairment but instead may reflect a speaker's attempt to find appropriate words in English. The example of the Vietnamese boy's narrative in this chapter reflects this point. His dysfluencies were not reflective of an impairment because his mother stated that he was fluent in Vietnamese. Instead, his dysfluencies appeared to reflect a limited proficiency in English; he was searching for the appropriate words to use in English. A native informant is the best source to determine whether dysfluencies were evident in speaker's native language. If they occur in both the first and second languages, an impairment would be suspected.

Intervention Considerations

The challenge for the professional is to preserve a child's cultural communication style and yet also enable the speaker to use a narrative style that is expected in school. This challenge is particularly poignant when two cultures are as contradictory with respect to communicative values as are the Japanese and European North American cultures. Conciseness is valued by the Japanese culture while elaboration is expected by teachers from European American backgrounds.

One way to approach this divergence is to distinguish between school and home discourse in a bilingual approach that has been previously described. Children can contrast the two styles while engaging in role-playing activities. A child can describe a past experience in a concise manner with related events (similar to a haiku) in the style expected in the community. The child can then describe that same event with much elaboration in the style expected in the school. A listener can pretend to be either a parent (expecting the concise version) or a teacher (expecting an elaborated version). In this approach, both communicative styles are valued and distinguished.

A child who cannot produce a concise two- or three-utterance form of narrative should be taught to do so. This type of narrative can be modeled and elicited both in the home and by the clinician. Once this structure has been mastered, more complete narrative structure can be elicited.

Some Asian children with language impairments may need to increase the informativeness dimension of narratives. The clinician can assist a speaker in elaborating discourse by asking directed questions about a child's experiences. Questions that elicit description and evaluation are "What did it look like?" and "How did you feel?" Informative narratives should be modeled and then elicited.

Stories from a child's culture are useful to secure a child's attention and interest regarding narrative discourse. Some relevant books are *Momotaro (The Peach Boy), Hanasaka Ji-San (The Old Man Who Made Trees Blossom)* (Sakade, 1958), and *Aekyng's Dream* (Paek, 1988). Children can retell the plots in these stories and then expand the stories with their own experiences. They can create personal narratives around similar events that others have related.

Professionals need to advise teachers about the cultural communicative values that members of some members of Asian communities may hold. Teachers should be encouraged to accept divergent communicative styles. In addition, they can encourage a more elaborate style by asking appropriate questions and modeling different genres.

In sum, the Asian community is diverse in the ethnic and linguistic groups that it reflects. We do not have sufficient information describing typical and impaired narrative discourse for all Asian communities. This chapter has presented information for assessment and intervention, based primarily on the Japanese community. Professionals need to recognize that narratives from Japanese children may be concise and consist of related episodes. These features represent a communicative style and not an impairment. A bilingual approach in intervention can be used to contrast a concise and an elaborated style. Children can be encouraged to use a more elaborated style in classroom settings.

Typical and Disordered Child Narration in Various Cultures

C. Clinical Applications

7

Assessment Guidelines for Children

In this chapter we present guidelines for the assessment of narrative discourse that are applicable to children across diverse cultures. The focus is on personal narratives because they are the most functional of the discourse genres we consider. Elicitation guidelines for personal narratives are presented in Chapter 1. First, however, we consider the variety of discourse genres that clinicians might want to use, from the simplest to the most difficult. We recommend, for example, that clinicians begin with personal narratives and then, if a child cannot complete a personal narrative, drop back to scripts or procedures. If a child cannot complete a script or procedure, clinicians might want to drop back to conversation, which is even easier because it is the most listener-supported genre. Note that although we have chosen to name our approach *narrative* assessment profile, we will proceed to demonstrate that the six dimensions we track are relevant to many different genres of discourse.

Genres of Discourse

The first task of assessing discourse capability is choosing from numerous genres of discourse. What follows is a brief typology of these genres, along with the virtues and drawbacks of each.

Genres That Are Easier Than Personal Narrative

Conversation.   Conversation consists of vocal exchanges between two or more participants. Conversation is the easiest genre because the listener can offer maximum support. For the same reason, it is not an optimum means of assessing more advanced children. The example that follows is an elicited conversation, one in which the interviewer has to ask many specific questions.

Example of conversation with a 9-year-old boy with specific language impairment (SLI) (from our files)

Adult: What are you going to do in Colorado?

Child: (1) . . . a lot of stuff, go to the mountains, throw rocks at the sea . . . (2) It's warm there (3) 'cuz it's summer there too, (4) but their only summer is only fourteen weeks . . . in the summer.

Adult: Who all is going?

Child: (5) . . . my sister, unless she doesn't want to go. (6) I don't want her to go.

Adult: So you're going by yourself?

Child: (7) No . . . my dad's . . . flying on a plane here (8) and then we're flying there . . .

Adult: You're going to fly to Colorado?

Child: (9) Mmmm hmmm . . . but we're gonna drive back.

Adult: Where are you going to get the car from?

Child: (10) My dad rents one from . . . his . . . his boss. (11) He's got all these . . . RVs. (12) Last time when we went, we drove back. (13) We drove over to Colorado (14) and we flew back (15) but this time we're flying there then back.

Adult: Tell me about the RV.

Child: (16) . . . It was . . . double times that it was supposed to be (17) and it had, it had a. . . . gas oven. (18) We had soup (19) and and I slept on the bed. (20) It was so high. (21) That's where I slept. (22) My sister slept on the couch, where I slept (23) and my dad slept um. . . . in the bed. (24) I slept in my area with a window (25) so you could see outside. (26) There was this one girl who stayed up. (27) She, she wanted to to go to get there faster instead of stopping. (28) My dad didn't stop, only for gas. (29) We got food. (30) We buyed about twenty bags of food. (31) We made like a lot of stops, (32) I mean, think about . . . California and back. (33) That's how far we went.

Some key points about this conversation are:

Topic Maintenance: Appropriate.

Event Sequencing: Not much in this excerpt; however, event sequencing is not necessarily an aspect of conversation.

Informativeness: Appropriate.

Referencing: Variable. The interviewer specifically asks "Who" and whether the narrator is going "by himself," so appropriate referencing is scaffolded. Comment 26 includes an unspecified reference: "this one girl."

Conjunctive Cohesion: Appropriate. A variety of conjunctions are used appropriately (e.g., 14, 15, 25).

Fluency: Inappropriate. There are hesitations (see . . . above in 1, 4, 5, 7, 9, among others) and repetitions are frequent (19, 27).

Intervention Goals.   The child's conversational discourse is adequate, but he needs help with narrative discourse. The clinician should attempt to increase the child's discourse coherence by having him construct short personal narratives, increase referencing in his narratives, and increase planning and self-monitoring of his personal narratives.

Scripts or Procedural Discourse.

A script consists of a brief description of a routine activity. It is characterized by the present tense, second-person perspective (e.g., *you,* although first- and third-person pronouns can be used if the activity is routine), explicit temporal sequencing, and simple sentences (Hudson & Shapiro, 1991). Three-year-olds can produce scriptal discourse for familiar events (Hudson & Shapiro, 1991). Scripts are elicited by asking a child a question about a routine activity. The general form of a prompt is "What do you do when you . . . (go to the doctor, go to a birthday party)?

One characteristic of scriptal discourse is that it is a relatively easy genre because it represents a form of discourse heavily structured by repeated experiences. The order of events is unambiguous, only one tense is involved, and there are few options for the speaker. It poses limited cognitive challenges because minimal effort is required to produce a clear message (Hudson & Shapiro, 1991). Scriptal discourse is appropriate for children who cannot produce long or complex texts. It enables professionals to obtain information regarding a simple text level form of discourse. The focus is on actions and ordering of events rather than descriptions, settings, feelings, and evaluations. The disadvantage of the genre is that scripts are too simple for more advanced children. Elicitation of scripts from advanced children does not provide enough information regarding textual features that are required in narrative, for example.

An example of a script elicited from an 8-year-old boy with specific language impairment (SLI) follows (from our files). He responded to the prompt "Tell me what you do at Burger King™."

> (1) We eat (2) and then sometimes we get like a little toy and in the . . . the in the bag. (3) We play with the little toy (4) um then we go back to our house (5) and then and then and then I go play with my friends.

Topic Maintenance: Appropriate. The speaker focuses all utterances on one topic.

Event Sequencing: Appropriate. Events are sequenced chronologically.

Informativeness: Inappropriate. There is missing information such as how to order, payment, how the child gets the toy, and how the food is removed from the table.

Referencing: Appropriate (note the use of *we*: this pronoun is acceptable because the speaker is describing a routine activity, his transition to *I* in utterance 5 departs from a script).

Conjunctive Cohesion: Appropriate. The speaker uses *and then* (2, 5) appropriately. Generally, more complex conjunctions are not found in scripts.

Fluency: Variable. Most utterances are fluent; however, there are repetitions in utterances 2 and 5.

Intervention Goals.   The clinician should focus on informativeness by encouraging the child to provide more details. Scripts can be varied in complexity by having a speaker describe a relatively routine procedure (e.g., checking out a library book) or an unfamiliar or abstract procedure (e.g., describing how to make a friend).

Personal Narrative

As we detailed in Chapter 1, personal narratives are descriptions of past events that have occurred to the narrator or someone else (Peterson & McCabe, 1983). Key features are past tense, use of setting, first and/or third person, explicit temporal sequencing (depending on the cultural values of this feature for the speaker), and inclusion of a high point (Labov, 1972; Peterson & McCabe, 1983). Chapter 1 gives details on how to elicit personal narratives successfully.

An advantage of a personal narrative is that this genre is complex, requiring much cognitive and pragmatic effort. A narrator must plan, sequence, and organize events without having been given a prior structure. A speaker must also determine how to describe the event so that the listener understands the message. This task requires social perspective taking; the listener must distinguish between what the listener already knows and what the listener needs to know and then relate a meaningful story. The complexity involved enables professionals to assess the discourse abilities of a speaker in organization and ordering of events, word retrieval, and fluency. Another advantage is its functionality. Speakers relate personal narratives frequently in their daily discourse. Five- to 7-year-old children use personal and vicarious narratives more than other types of discourse in their conversations with peers (Preece, 1987). Narratives are also commonly used in educational settings (see Chapter 2).

The complexity of the personal narrative genre can also be a disadvantage. Some children with language impairments will not be able to produce a personal narrative because of the cognitive and discourse challenges it poses. For such children, a simpler discourse genre, such as conversation or scripts, will need to be evaluated.

Genres That May Be More Difficult Than Personal Narrative

Prompted Story Retelling.   This genre is present on several language assessment tests (e.g., the *CELF*, Semel, Wiig, & Secord, 1995; the *Goldman Fristoe*, Goldman &

Fristoe, 2000) and requires the speaker to repeat a story to a listener. It is a highly structured task that does not require creativity by a speaker.

Three procedures have been used to elicit story retelling. In one procedure, the clinician tells a story to a child and asks the child to repeat or retell the story. A second procedure requires the child to view a videotape and then to retell the story. A third procedure has the child view a wordless picture book and retell the story. The stimuli in this case are pictures, which differs from the first procedure. It is considered to be story retelling because the pictures depict a preconceived story, meaning that the child is required to retell the story illustrated in the pictures rather than to create one. Whether the pictures are viewed by the child during the task will vary with examiner.

In story retelling, sometimes the child shares knowledge of the story with the clinician, sometimes not. In a shared context, the clinician and the child both hear (or view) the same story. The child repeats known or shared information back to the adult, which many children find strange and which can spur summarization from some children and embellishment (to keep from boring the listener) from others. In an unshared context, the child retells the story to a listener who has not participated in the initial part of the retelling task. The child presents new information to a listener. Stories are more complete and longer in an unshared context (Liles, 1987; Menig-Peterson, 1978).

The advantage of story retelling is that it is associated with a relatively high interscorer reliability rate because the original text is available to the scorer. Fewer dysfluencies and word retrieval deficits are evident in this genre than in spontaneous stories because the material has been presented to the child (Merritt & Liles, 1989). Length of retold stories is greater than that of spontaneous fictional stories because the task is easier (Merritt & Liles, 1989). Retelling a story is a relatively simple task because events do not need to be ordered; they are already sequenced. Thus, 4-year-old children should be able to do this task (Hedberg & Westby, 1993; McKeogh, 1987).

A disadvantage of story retelling is that it is not a demanding or sensitive task (Hedberg & Westby, 1993; Merritt & Liles, 1989). Knowledge of story structure will not be revealed in this genre because the story has already been provided for the child. Deficits in fluency, word retrieval, and event sequencing may not be evident with this task.

The following story was used by Culatta, Page, and Ellis (1983, p. 73):

(1) Tommy was 5 years old. (2) His birthday was coming soon. (3) He wanted a puppy for his birthday (4) but his mother said that he was too little to take care of it. (5) Tommy didn't think that he was too little. (6) He decided to show his parents that he was big enough to have a puppy. (7) He bought a leash and dog food. (8) He told his parents that he would always take care of the puppy. (9) When his birthday came, Tommy had a party. (10) Five of his friends came to his house. (11) They played games, ate animal crackers and cookies. (12) Tommy opened his presents. (13) He got a GI Joe, a fire truck, some comic books, and a baseball bat. (14) He liked the presents (15) but he was disappointed (16) because he didn't get a puppy.

(17) All of Tommy's friends were getting ready to go home, when his daddy brought out another present for him to open. (18) Inside was a little black puppy. (19) Tommy was really happy (20) because he got the present he wanted. (21) Tommy promised to take good care of the puppy. (22) The end.[1]

The following story retelling was elicited from an 11-year-, 3-month-old boy with SLI (from our files). The numbers of the utterances in the original story are presented at the end of each utterance.

(1) One day Tommy wanted a puppy [3] (2) but his parents said that he's too young to have a puppy [4] (3) so he showed his parents that he could take care of the puppy by showing them a leash and.....................a leash and...........a...........uh dish [7] (4) so his party came [9]. (5) Um his five friends came to the party [10]. (6) They ate........... animal crackers, chips, and um...punch [11] (7) but he got a GI Joe, a fire truck, some comic books and a...............cards [13] (8) so his but his friends were about to leave [17] (9) but his dad come with a present for him to open [17]. (10) Inside was a black puppy and um...........................[18]. (11) He said that he that he will promise to take care of the puppy [18]. (12) The end [19].

Topic Maintenance: Appropriate. All the utterances are focused around a central theme.

Event Sequencing: Appropriate. Comparison of the order of events in the original story to the order of events in the retold story reveals that the child's story is in the same chronological order.

Informativeness: Inappropriate. Information is missing about orientation (original utterances 1 and 2), internal feelings, and reactions (original utterances: 5, 6, 14–16, 19–20).

Referencing: Appropriate. The speaker identifies the main characters (e.g., parents and friends) and objects; his pronoun usage in 6, 7, and 9 refers to referents appropriately identified in previous utterances; the pronoun *he* in utterance 18 is understood by the context. There was no opportunity for spontaneous use of referents because of the nature of this genre; all referent information was presented in the story.

Conjunctive Cohesion: Variable. *But* is used correctly to denote adversative meaning in 2, while *so* is used correctly to denote causality in 3. Pragmatic use of *so* in 4 to denote slight change of focus is apt. On the other hand *but* in 7, *so . . . but* in 8, and *but* in 9 are neither semantically nor pragmatically apt.

Fluency: Inappropriate. There are several lengthy pauses (6, 7, 10).

[1]Culatta, B., Page, J., & Ellis, G. (1983). Story retelling as a communicative performance screening tool. *Language, Speech, and Hearing Services in Schools, 14*, 73. © American Speech-Language-Hearing Association. Reprinted by permission.

Intervention Goals. We would not use this genre as a basis for intervention because it is not functional communication. After children master personal narratives, clinicians can use story retelling as one aspect of an intervention hierarchy in order to enable children to produce a text. If this genre is incorporated in therapy, the unshared context should be used since it maximizes discourse performance.

Spontaneous Fiction Retelling. A type of retelling that falls between prompted retelling, just described, and spontaneous fiction that follows consists of describing a familiar movie or book plot. Clinicians can simply ask a child to tell about a movie or book with which the speaker (and, preferably, the clinician) is familiar. An advantage of this type of narrative is that it has less structure than prompted retelling and is more spontaneous than the other forms. It is more structured than personal narratives, in that the story was already composed by someone else. The fact that this type of fiction has an existing structure (either with a prompt or a description of a familiar story) may enable some children to show abilities beyond the simple genres discussed previously. The disadvantage is that it may be too difficult for some children.

An example of a fictional retelling of the movie *Poltergeist* follows. A 9-year-old child with SLI described this movie in response to the prompt "Tell me about *Poltergeist*; I haven't seen the movie yet."

> (1) That and the g . . . girl comes up and (2) he's the going on and off, on off (3) 'cuz there's like these Martians in the TV and um and (4) the girl goes, "Ah." (5) She goes, she goes, "They're here" (6) and um next thing hear a noise going "poof" like a tornado (7) and wakes up (8) and then the girl's still standing there and the TV. (9) It was really a cute movie (10) and you should see it. . . . (11) The girl monster was eating the boy and was like a tree (12) and they boy was . . . (13) This clown was about to choke him like it's like a doll (14) but it's coming to life (15) and um this tree, he was looking at the tree (16) 'cuz it look like it had a mouth (17) then when the tornado come, it had a mouth (18) and it ate him up. (19) Yeah, but they got him out . . . (20) All blood all over him (21) and they hadta wash him off. . . . (22) You know what? (23) The girl's just standing here with (makes a facial expression of astonishment) looking (24) then she was just standing there.

Topic Maintenance: Appropriate. All utterances focus on the movie, including the two direct comments to the listener (utterances 9 and 10).

Event Sequencing: Inappropriate. This type of narrative is called leapfrogging because the speaker jumps around and leaves so many key events out that someone who has not seen the movie would make very little sense of what was said. Note that the description of the girl is presented in the beginning (utterances 1, 8) and at the end (utterances 23–24). The other events do not appear to be described in chronological order.

Informativeness: Inappropriate. There is not enough information for the listener to understand the story. The speaker does not provide details about the setting, characters, main events, and resolution. There is also no ending.

Referencing: Inappropriate. The speaker has not sufficiently identified the characters (e.g., the girl in utterance 1; the boy, utterance, 11; the clown, utterance 13). Pronouns do not have sufficient prior identification (e.g., *it* utterance 14; *he* utterance 15; *him* utterances 18, 20, 21; and *they* in utterances, 19, 21). There is one erroneous referent, *he* for *it* in utterance 2.

Conjunctive Cohesion: Appropriate. The speaker uses *and*, "cuz," and *but* appropriately for semantic conjunction.

Fluency: Variable. There are segments of fluent productions (utterances 3–10 and 13–19). There are repetitions that may be used by the speaker for emphasis (utterance 2). But there are also pauses (utterances, 10, 19, 21) and one abandoned utterance (12).

Intervention Goals.   The speaker needs to improve most aspects of narration. We would begin with an easier form of discourse, such as scripts and procedures, in order for him to master basic event sequencing and informativeness. We do not know whether there would be generalization to a more complex form, such a fictional retelling. We doubt it because of the complexity of the latter genre. We would then ask him to tell a personal narrative, and work with him to ensure that he was capable of telling a fully developed one. If, after the speaker developed the ability to tell an adequate personal narrative, fictional storytelling were also a goal (due to classroom requirements), we would proceed with relatively simple fictional stories with few characters and events. Gradually, we could increase length and complexity by adding optional elements, additional characters, and internal states.

Spontaneous Fiction.   This genre consists of two forms. One type is production of a fictional story, usually with a prompt (e.g., Nicole was lost in the woods. She found a house. What happened to her?). Another type involves asking the child to make up a story without an initial story stem.

Length and complexity will vary depending upon the abilities of the narrator. This genre is more complex than scripts or procedural discourse because there is less structure given to the child. The child must develop the narrative from the beginning.

The features of this genre are setting, characters, temporal sequencing of events, problem resolution of a situation, and ending (Hudson & Shapiro, 1991; Stein & Glenn, 1979). There can be optional features that serve to elaborate a story such as additional characters, inclusion of internal states, different perspectives of the characters, and embedded events.

This genre is difficult for children with language disorders because of the absence of provided structure; that is, speakers need to develop their own organization and plan their message (Purcell & Liles, 1992).

Issues Pertaining to Multicultural Narrative Assessment

The purpose of this section is to address issues that pertain to the assessment of narrative discourse that are relevant for speakers from multicultural backgrounds.

1. *Ask about, don't assume, cultural background, especially language exposure.* Professionals should not assume that they can determine a child's culture by looking at the child or even by hearing that the child seems to have a typical American accent. Recall the Haitian child whose narratives opened Chapter 1. Numerous children whose discourse may be very much influenced by the culture of origin of their parents look and sound like children whose families have been in the country for decades, if not centuries. Nonetheless, their discourse often differs upon close scrutiny, which is a key point of this book. Professionals should always inquire as to a child's cultural background. We recommend asking the questions in Box 7.1.

BOX 7.1 • *Determining Child's Cultural/Linguistic Background*

1. What is the language background of people who live with your child? Include both parents, brothers and sisters, grandparents, babysitters, and anyone else who spends a lot of time interacting with your child.
2. It is important that adults interact with children in the language with which they are most familiar and in which they feel most comfortable. What language do the people who spend a lot of time with your child use with your child?
3. How long have these people been in the United States?
4. Some people like children to talk a lot about the experiences they remember, other people prefer children to be brief. When you ask your child about a past experience, how much do you want him or her to talk? What are you most interested in hearing about?

2. *Test results versus narrative abilities.* Formal testing is a basic component of assessment protocols used by speech-language pathologists. Test results are needed to justify a child's placement in remedial services and to demonstrate improvement and treatment efficacy. Test data do not always reflect narrative abilities, however, and this discrepancy is especially likely in the case of children for whom English is a second language, children for whom tests have often not been sufficiently normed. For example, a child who is inattentive, distractible, or poorly motivated may not do well on a standardized test. However, this same child may show appropriate narrative discourse. In contrast, a child may perform within age limits on a test but perform poorly on a narrative discourse task because the latter is more demanding and challenging. In short, behavior elicited on a structured test could differ from performance found in an unstructured context, such as narrative discourse.

An example of the difference between performance in two contexts is evident with the child below. He is a bilingual 10-year-old Spanish-speaking child who failed two standardized language tests, one in English and one in Spanish. He provided the following narrative in English:

Adult: Have you ever been to the hospital?

Child: My friend has. He has a broken arm.

Adult: Tell me about it.

Child: Some other kid, he was fighting with him. Then he dropped his arm and he sat on it and he broke it.

Adult: He broke it?

Child: And they had to put a cast on him and he was crying until he went to the hospital.

Adult: What else happened?

Child: Um they they told his mom and that kid got in trouble. He's grounded forever uh until they take the cast off him. Then he could start playing with his friends but he can't go to his house and his dad doesn't want him there.

This child produced a well-organized and coherent narrative. He sequences events and provides a consequence to his story. He does well with the six dimensions of NAP. In spite of poor test scores, this child is able to produce a coherent narrative.

In other cases, students may pass standardized tests and yet flounder in producing narrative. In fact, Biddle, McCabe, and Bliss (1996) document the case of one such individual with traumatic brain injury who was struggling in school writing assignments despite having passed a battery of standardized tests. Her narration revealed the problems that made writing so difficult for her even though the tests of vocabulary, syntax, and so on did not reveal problems.

3. *Interpreters.* Interpreters may be used in situations in which professionals do not have sufficient knowledge of a child's first language. The use of interpreters in assessment can be controversial. While they have knowledge of a speaker's first language, they are not trained to assess language behavior. If they must be used, interpreters should be trained to carefully provide the clinician with the exact utterances that a speaker has produced. It is a common tendency for some adults to fill in missing words or correct the grammar of children. Interpreters need to be trained not to unconsciously correct a child's production when interpreting the child's utterances.

4. *Judgments by members of a child's community.* Differences in cultural background influence the interpretation and judgment of the adequacy of narratives. Michaels (1991) showed that African American and European North American judges differed in their assessment of the quality of the narratives produced by an African American child. The evaluations ranged from coherent to jumbled. We had a similar experience with different interpretations of a narrative as shown in the sample that follows. It was elicited from a 4-year, 7-month-old African American child who was diagnosed as language impaired:

Adult: I used to have a dog. He was big and brown. I really liked him. One day he ran away and never came back. Have you ever had a pet run away?

Child: No . . . when I get some pets, they be, they be using it in our house.

Adult: Uh huh.

Child: Because we be taking them outside and they don't be move because they don't need to move. Ain't no need to use the bathroom though.

Adult: Can you tell me more?

Child: When they come in there, they use it. We be going outside quickest. We be running outs . . . out the door.

Adult: You be running out the door?

Child: Ummmm. We be on the door and we run out through it and our pappy in the back uh and she . . . uh he use it. He got a big cage for all of them.

Adult: A cage for one of them?

Child: Uh huh, we got lots of dogs.

Adult: You got lots of dogs?

Child: Once when we have five dogs and none ran away.

Adult: You have five dogs and none ran away?

Child: Then we played with them. We brought them some chew toys and they chew them when they hungry. That's the end of my story.

Two different interpretations were made of this narrative. An experienced African American speech-language pathologist understood this child's narrative. Specifically, she explained, the child related that he did not experience a pet running away from home. Instead, he described difficulties in training the family dogs to go to the bathroom outside. Because the dogs could not be trained, the father put them outside in a big cage. The narrator and his siblings had fun playing with those dogs. They bought toys for the dogs, who chewed these toys when they were hungry.

On the other hand, two European North American professionals, who are experienced with narratives, viewed this narrative as exhibiting somewhat reduced coherence. The meaning of the child's narrative was not clear to them.

This example highlights the impact of cultural influences on the judgment of narrative coherence. Clinicians may make the same types of misperceptions when assessing the narratives of children from other different cultures. For example, clinicians might mistake the conciseness of Japanese narratives for an impairment in referencing or informativeness, specifically elaboration, when the narrative may be reflecting the culture of the speaker. Children may come to school without knowing expectations for the types of narratives expected in an academic environment (Gutiérrez-Clellen, 1996). Their narratives may reflect such a lack of knowledge and experience of what is expected of them rather than a narrative deficiency per se (Gutiérrez-Clellen, 1996). For this reason, the quality of narratives needs to be judged by members of a speaker's community.

Analysis of Narrative Discourse

We have described different approaches to the analyses of narratives (Hedberg & Westby, 1993; Hughes, McGillivray, & Schmidek, 1997; Chapter 1). In this chapter we will focus on two efficient procedures that will enable professionals to obtain a comprehensive view of a child's abilities.

Narrative Structure: Phase I

Once a narrative sample has been transcribed, a high-point analysis can be completed in order to describe the structure of a child's narrative (McCabe & Rollins, 1994). Note that this phase is most appropriate for children from African American or European North American homes, or children from other backgrounds for whom English is the first language. The purpose of this analysis is to identify discourse-level abilities with respect to overall narrative structure, which also requires a close look at the basic components of narration (which will be required for Phase II, as well). The clinician places a narrative into one of several different categories that have been described from a developmental framework (Peterson & McCabe, 1983). A brief summary of the categories is presented in Box 7.2.

McCabe and Rollins (1994) suggested a series of questions for clinicians to answer to determine the type of structure a child's narrative represents. Table 7.1 illustrates a format that can be used (McCabe & Rollins, 1994, p. 49).

BOX 7.2 • *Phase 1: High-Point Structure*

Two-event narrative: a sequence that involves two actions; generally produced by children under 4 years of age.

Leapfrog narrative: a narrative about a single experience that consists of more than two events that are not presented in logical or chronological order and that is characterized by omission of salient information; generally produced by 4-year-old children with typical language development.

End-at-high-point narrative: a narrative that includes all of the necessary information except the consequence or resolution of an experience; generally produced by 5-year-old children.

Classic narrative: a narrative that contains all of the necessary information for a coherent story; generally produced by 6-year-old North American European and African American children with typical language development.

Chronological narrative: a narrative that is characterized by lists of actions that are not causally related, generally produced by children of all ages and even adults. A typical example is a travel itinerary.

Miscellaneous narrative: a narrative that cannot be placed in one of the above categories.

TABLE 7.1 *Phase 1: High-Point Scoring Guidelines*

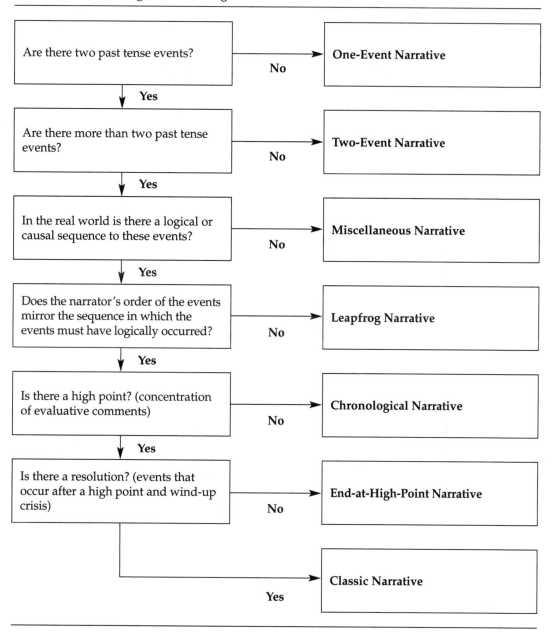

McCabe, A., & Rollins, P.R. (1994). Assessment of preschool narrative skills. *American Journal of Speech-Language Pathology: A Journal of Clinical Practice, 3,* 45–56. © American Speech-Language-Hearing Association. Reprinted by permission.

The narrative produced by the child with specific language impairment in Chapter 3 will be used to show an example of high-point analysis. The answer to the first three questions in Table 7.1 is yes. That is to say, (1) yes, there are two past-tense events; (2) yes, there are more than two past-tense events; and (3) yes, in the real world we have every reason to believe there was a chronological order to those events. However, the answer to the fourth question is no, the narrator's order of the events does not mirror the sequence in which the events must have logically occurred. Thus, his narrative represents a leapfrogging structure; the child skipped around in his description of events and omitted critical information. He began by talking about the hospital and then described his bike accident and then returned to the hospital situation. It should be noted that leapfrogging narratives are used by some 4-year-old children with typical language development. Older children should be able to sequence events. Additional examples of high-point analysis are presented in Peterson and McCabe (1983; McCabe & Rollins, 1994).

Narrative Structure: Phase II

The second step in narrative assessment is to identify the specific dimensions that are appropriately and inappropriately used. In this way, a profile of abilities and deficits can be used as a basis of intervention. The narrative analysis profile (described in Chapter 1) was developed to meet this purpose. We have used it to describe the narratives elicited from speakers throughout this book.

Following are guidelines for implementing the NAP:

1. Score discourse according to whether it is appropriate, variable, inappropriate, or in need of further study (see Chapter 1).
2. Establish profiles of strengths and weaknesses among dimensions. Children with language disorders do not exhibit a homogeneous grouping of symptoms. Different patterns of impairment of narrative abilities are identifiable for individuals bearing the same diagnosis despite the fact that general tendencies for people with that diagnosis exist and have been documented (Miranda, McCabe, & Bliss, 1998). For example, one child with specific language impairment may be characterized by impairments in topic maintenance, event sequencing, and informativeness with strengths in conjunctive cohesion and fluency; another child with SLI might exhibit excessive dysfluencies and referencing impairments with strength in the other dimensions (Miranda, McCabe, & Bliss, 1998). One frequent pattern of children and adults with traumatic brain injury is impairments in fluency and informativeness, as well as substantial redundancy, although event sequencing is appropriate (Biddle, McCabe, & Bliss, 1996).
3. Use a form such as the Narrative Assessment Protocol on page 121 to identify different profiles of narrative ability. This form enables clinicians to assess narrative abilities efficiently.

In Chapter 1 (p. 41), we demonstrated how to use the Narrative Assessment Profile. At the end of this chapter (p. 122), we use NAP to score narrative discourse produced by a child with a language impairment. This child showed considerable impairments in topic maintenance, event sequencing, informativeness, and fluency. He was variable with respect to referencing and conjunctive cohesion. This protocol enables us to see the broad reductions in his discourse coherence with respect to narratives.

Working for the First Time with Children from a Cultural Group Unknown to You

The United States is rich in the variety of individuals who immigrate here, so many cultures have not been researched carefully. What should educators and clinicians do when they confront a child from a culture about which they know very little? We recommend that educators and clinicians proceed much as researchers do at the outset of an exploration:

1. Keep an open mind about the quality of the narratives you hear or read.
2. Look for patterns in those narratives; do *not* look first to see how well these narratives match our cultural expectations for a good story (embodied in Phase 1, high-point scoring in Table 7.1).
3. Seek help from full participants in the child's culture.
4. Perhaps expand your definition of what makes a good story. Use what you have learned about other cultures to assist you in this.

We put those principles to work consistently. Recently, for example, David Colby, Keith Erwin, and the first author (Colby & Erwin, 2001) began studying the personal narratives of 6- to 10-year-old Cambodian English bilingual children. The children attend a trilingual education program, where instruction is offered in Kmer, Spanish, and English. We were hampered by many factors, including the lack of a collaborator from the Cambodian community, access to a small number of children varying in age, and limited resources. We elicited narratives in English using the procedure outlined in Chapter 1. The Cambodian children were not inclined to be talkative, but all contributed several narratives and seemed eager to do so. Among the best of the thirty narratives we obtained from ten Cambodian American children were the following from two different boys:

> **Narrative: 9-year-old Cambodian boy (from our files)**
> **Interviewer:** . . . I cut my knee pretty bad. Have you ever hurt yourself?
>
> **Child:** Yes. (1) Once I ran up the stairs so fast that I slipped (2) and I hit my leg. (3) And one time I went down a big hill, (4) and I made a jump, (5) and then I landed and crashed into a car. (6) And once at the skate park, I went down the hill and crashed into some boards, (7) and then I crashed into my fence, (8) and I flew off my bike.
>
> **Interviewer:** What happened after that?
>
> **Child:** (9) I had a lot of Band-Aids on myself.

Narrative: 10-year-old Cambodian boy (from our files)

Interviewer: . . . I cut my knee pretty bad. Have you ever hurt yourself?

Child: Yes. (1) When I was riding my skateboards, I rode it down the hill, (2) and I was going into the street, (3) So I just let it go, (4) And the car ran over the skateboard.

Interviewer: What happened after that?

Child: (5) I was so mad, (6) So I said (with emphasis denoted by italics), *"You should watch where you're riding!"* (7) And the last time when I was riding my bike, I rode down the hill, (8) I lost control, (9) so I stopped the brake and turned, (10) and I went all the way into the trashcan.

Interviewer: . . . What happened?

Child: (11) I had to go to the doctor.

These were two of the most fluent of the thirty narratives we collected, and you will note that both are concise narrations of two- or three-injury experiences. We were reminded of Japanese children's narration in this regard. Note that neither one exhibits a classic narrative structure (Phase I), but because we knew so little about Cambodian storytelling, we had already decided to set that analysis aside.

We have developed a number of hypotheses about Cambodian storytelling preferences. We suspect that, like all the other cultures the first author has studied to date except for the European North American culture, Cambodians prefer narratives about several related experiences. That is, their notion of topic development would be quite different from the European North American one. Event sequencing is logical in both narratives, so we suspect that is an emphasis, at least for children. Informativeness is, as always, a key issue. Here we again are inclined to believe that Cambodians value conciseness over extensive elaboration. Both narratives contain action and evaluation, but not much description. We wonder whether this is a value of Cambodian narration or due to the fact that these are child narrators speaking English as a second language. Referencing is appropriate in both narratives, with the slight exception that a car is introduced as "the car" the first time in the second narrative. Conjunctions are used aptly in both. Both are fluently produced. We look forward to hearing more from such children.

To summarize the main points about assessment, clinicians need to consider the cultural and linguistic backgrounds and the communicative values of children's communities. Narrative discourse should be evaluated with respect to high-point analysis, in some cases, and the narrative assessment profile (NAP) in any case. The NAP is useful for comparing a child's strengths and weaknesses and identifying directions for intervention.

NARRATIVE ASSESSMENT PROTOCOL

Name of Client: _____ **Date of Birth:** _____

Narrative Elicitor: _____ **Cultural/Linguistic Background:** _____

Narrative Aspect	Appropriate, Variable, Inappropriate, Needs Further Study	Description of Narrative Discourse
Topic Maintenance		
Event Sequencing		
Informativeness		
Referencing		
Conjunctive Cohesion		
Fluency		

Conclusions and recommendations: _____

_____

A completed NAP will be found on the next page.

NARRATIVE ASSESSMENT PROTOCOL

Name of Client: _____ **Date of Birth:** <u>(9 years 3 months)</u>

Narrative Eliticor: _____ **Cultural/Linguistic Background:** <u>European North American</u>

Narrative Aspect	*Appropriate, Variable, Inappropriate, Needs Further Study*	*Description of Narrative Discourse*
Topic Maintenance	Inappropriate	Intermingling of topics
Event Sequencing	Inappropriate	Leapfrogging narrative
Informativeness	Inappropriate	Insufficient information Reduced elaboration Minimal description Uses action
Referencing	Variable	Some omissions and unspecified; family members identified correctly
Conjunctive Cohesion	Variable	Mostly has appropriate use of semantic and pragmatic functions; two errors
Fluency	Inappropriate	Excessive dysfluencies of false starts, internal corrections, repetitions, fillers

Conclusions and recommendations: <u>Impaired narrative abilities for his age. Intervention with goals to improve topic maintenance, event sequencing, and informativeness.</u>

8

Intervention Guidelines for Children

In this chapter, we present guidelines for intervention that are applicable to children from all cultures. The chapter includes indications of the need for intervention, selection of intervention goals, approaches to intervention, general intervention guidelines, specific procedures, programming for classrooms, and parent programs.

Indications for Intervention

Is there a need for intervention at the narrative level? This question can be difficult to answer because normative data concerning narrative abilities for speakers from many different cultural and linguistic backgrounds are not currently available. Furthermore, narratives vary to some degree in their length and content depending upon topic, listener, and setting (Peterson & McCabe, 1983). Standardized elicitation procedures are not common. Clinicians need to make their own evaluations in narrative assessment, as we have indicated in the previous chapter. If professionals practice, they will achieve reliability and can then determine whether a speaker needs intervention for narrative abilities. In our research, for example, two raters achieved extremely high correlations on independent ratings of data using the narrative assessment profile (NAP). Specifically, the correlation between numbers of explicit propositions and between numbers of implicit propositions exceeded .94, alpha less than .001, for children with specific language impairment, traumatic brain injury, and typical language development (Bliss, McCabe, & Miranda, 1998; Miranda, McCabe, & Bliss, 1998). *Impaired narration* is defined as reduced discourse coherence with deficits in one or more dimensions of narration.

Clinicians will also determine the necessity for intervention based on information that is provided by a child's significant others (e.g., parents, teachers, and peers). Some questions that professionals can ask the people who interact with the child are presented in Box 8.1.

BOX 8.1 • *Questions to Ask Parents, Teachers, and Peers about a Child's Discourse Performance (adapted by second author from Damico, 1985; Paul, 2001).*

1. Do you understand what the child is trying to convey when she or he tells you about something that has happened?
2. Are there many hesitations, pauses, and repetitions in the child's utterances?
3. When talking about something, does the child leave out important details, present too much information, or repeat information?
4. Does the child switch topics often?
5. Does the child identify the people, places, and objects that are mentioned?
6. Does the child talk for too long a time?
7. Does the child present information out of order?
8. Does the child provide accurate information?

Selection of Intervention Goals

One intervention goal is to preserve the narrative style that a speaker uses in the community. One prominent African American educator makes a point about African American dialect that is relevant here—Delpit (Perry & Delpit, 1998, pp. 17–18) points out that "despite good intentions, constant correction seldom has the desired effect. Such correction increases cognitive monitoring of speech, thereby making talking difficult." Professionals are far more likely to be successful if working *with* the grain of wood—*with* the skills a child brings to school—instead of against them. Repeatedly devaluing what skills a child does have and has learned from beloved parents is likely to result in alienation rather than improvement. In fact, the first author has advocated and outlined some important aspects of a serious multicultural literature-based program of instruction in *Chameleon Readers: Teaching Children to Appreciate All Kinds of Good Stories* (McCabe, 1996). There are many compelling reasons that all children would benefit from such a program, including an ability to eventually comprehend Nobel-Prize-winning world literature, increased understanding of all kinds of peers with whom someday they will work, and decreased racism.

However, also following the arguments put forth by many minority educators (see Perry & Delpit, 1998), we suggest introducing a narrative style that is used and expected in schools in order to enable a child to perform successfully in that environment. Therefore, narratives that incorporate at least two events and optimal performance on the six dimensions of the NAP will be the goal.

Narrative Structure

Before a professional can facilitate narrative content, appropriate basic narration should be elicited. Initially a child should be able to provide at least two events in a narrative. Narrative length should be gradually increased. The goal is to facilitate classic narrative structure because that is the style of narrative increasingly required on high-stakes testing, among other places. This type of narrative includes a setting, high point, evaluation, and resolution.

Narrative Content

The concept of triage is applicable to the choices professionals make in selecting appropriate targets for intervention (Bliss, McCabe, & Miranda, 1998). The six narrative dimensions of NAP reflect general and specific domains. The more general dimensions are topic maintenance, event sequencing, and informativeness. They have a broad effect on discourse coherence and should be targeted early if impaired.

The more specific dimensions of discourse are referencing and fluency, which are more limited in their impact on discourse coherence. Sometimes they only affect the coherence of one or two utterances. These dimensions should be secondary goals because their impact is restricted.

Conjunctive cohesion should be relegated to the final stages of intervention. Children with and without impairments frequently use *and* and *and then* for their narratives (Peterson & McCabe, 1987). Additional conjunctions can be added after the other narrative dimensions have been improved.

Specific Approaches to Intervention

Didactic Intervention

This approach is designed to teach specific aspects of discourse. The rationale is that children with language impairments have not learned language spontaneously and they need to learn the rules of discourse with a structured approach (Naremore, Densmore, & Harmon, 1995). The clinician serves as a teacher rather than a conversational partner and focuses on specific rules of discourse and their implementation (Naremore, Densmore, & Harmon, 1995). For example, topic maintenance is elicited by teaching the concept of topic and emphasizing the need to stay on one topic while talking (Naremore, Densmore, & Harmon, 1995). Children identify topics that are maintained and others that diverge from a central theme by observing videotapes of speakers. They are also taught how to indicate topic shifts. They enact scripts and engage in role playing as a means of learning to use the rules that they have been taught (Naremore, Densmore, & Harmon, 1995).

The didactic approach is useful because specific information is highlighted through rules. It can be effective for some school-aged children (Naremore, Densmore, & Harmon, 1995). However, for many it may be too abstract. Some children do not have the metalinguistic, metapragmatic, and cognitive skills to understand the concept of discourse rules. Furthermore, generalization from rule learning to spontaneous discourse may be difficult for some children.

Discourse-Based Intervention

In this approach, narrative coherence is improved implicitly through functional communicative and interactive tasks (Bliss, 1993; Owens, 1999). This approach is based on the rationale that children with language impairments will generalize their new discourse skills if functional communicative contexts and procedures are implemented (Bliss, 1993; Owens, 1999). The clinician serves as a conversational partner rather than a teacher.

An example of a discourse-based procedure would be to have the professional elicit appropriate topic maintenance in a narrative. Instead of telling the child to maintain a topic (a discourse rule), the adult would signal to the child that some utterances deviated from a topic by asking contingent queries or using verbal redirection. Adults pose discourse-based *contingent queries* that help the speaker to return to the main topic. They signal that a communication breakdown has occurred because topic maintenance was not achieved. The professional asks questions such as "Who did it?" or "What happened to Sally?" as a means of enabling the speaker to return to the original topic.

Verbal redirection can also be used; the adult asks a question and answers it and then asks a child the question again (Lucas, 1980), as in the following hypothetical exchange:

Clinician: Where did you go yesterday?

Child: Mommy bought a new coat.

Clinician: You went to the store with your mother?

Child: Yes.

Clinician: You went to the store with your mother. Where did you go yesterday?

Child: To the store.

This approach is expected to facilitate generalization of behaviors because functional communication contexts and discourse-based strategies are used as part of the direct intervention, rather than being contexts to which the intervention is supposed to generalize. However, some children may profit from more explicit structure and specific teaching. Professionals should adapt their approach to suit particular children.

Combined Didactic and Discourse-Based Approach

This approach combines both of the approaches previously described. Children are not taught rules but are instructed to talk about an event or to "tell me as much information as you can." Professionals direct children in their communicative attempts in a less structured manner than is used in the didactic approach; however, they highlight certain discourse behaviors. Discourse-based techniques and modeling approaches are used to elicit narrative coherence.

For example, to increase topic maintenance, the professional might model a brief narrative or a segment of a narrative as a means of focusing on a passage in which all utterances are related to one theme. The professional would then ask the child to tell a narrative about one occurrence and would use contingent queries and verbal redirection techniques to assist the child in this process. The steps of this approach, developed by the second author, can be summarized in the acronym DIME, as in Box 8.2:

BOX 8.2 • *DIME: Combined Didactic and Discourse-Based Intervention*

1. *D = Discourse Attempt*
   The child attempts a narrative. If it is inappropriate, steps 2–4 are carried out.
2. *I = Identification*
   The clinician asks directed questions in order to identify the aspects of the narrative that were not appropriate. The questions might function to redirect the child to the original topic or introduce referents that have not been previously identified. They might also function to provide additional information that was missing. If the child added extraneous material to a narrative about a hospital visit, for example, the adult would use verbal redirection to enable the child to return to the original topic.
3. *M = Model*
   The professional models the complete narrative or segments of the narrative to focus on the aspects that were originally inappropriate. The adult would model corrected or expanded portions of the child's attempt in order to demonstrate, through discourse, how to produce an oral text in which utterances all relate to a topic.
4. *E = Elicited Production*
   The professional asks the child to produce the original or a similar narrative. This production may be coconstructed, with the professional and the speaker both relating parts of the narrative. Elicited production may also consist of unassisted narrative attempts.

General Intervention Guidelines

1. Preserve a speaker's cultural style and add other options. Silva and McCabe (1996, p. 31) advocated, "We have to tell children from non-European backgrounds that their language and culture are unique and wonderful but they have to learn how to master another set of rules."
2. Incorporate a speaker's community into intervention by including prominent cultural features in discourse activities, such as discussing food and holidays (Kayser, 1995). Use relevant literature, stories, and folklore that are familiar to a child.

3. Consider a second-language learning approach in which different discourse styles are contrasted. Efforts must be made to treat both discourse styles as acceptable and worthy. A bidialectal approach will succeed only if both styles are appreciated for their communicative value (Campbell, 1996).

4. Use discourse hierarchies. One hierarchy involves progressing from simple to more complex genres. For example, as we noted in the preceding chapter on assessment, relatively easy tasks involve describing simple procedures or routine events (e.g., scripts or procedures), such as making a peanut butter and jelly sandwich. More complex discourse tasks involve describing a baseball or basketball game (e.g., a harder procedural discourse) or an experience (e.g., personal narrative).

   Another hierarchy involves length; shorter narratives should be elicited before longer ones. Discourse complexity involves other, more specific hierarchies, such as adding more actions and participants in an event; increasing the displacement of time or location; and including mental states, motivation, and inferences in a narrative (Norris & Hoffman, 1993).

5. Incorporate a variety of narrative genres to promote discourse flexibility, including fictional stories (either spontaneously constructed ones or descriptions of familiar books or movies) and personal and vicarious narratives.

6. Enable children to tell narratives in different contexts, such as formal situations (e.g., classrooms) and more informal contexts (e.g., recess).

7. Use meaningful communication by enabling the child to convey new information to a listener. Speakers are inherently motivated to convey novel and interesting information (Hudson & Shapiro, 1991).

Specific Intervention Procedures for Narrative Structure (High Point)

One intervention goal is to enable children to produce a classic narrative with at least two events and a setting, high point, and resolution. In order to enable children to produce at least two-event narratives, clinicians can show them pictures with a single character performing different actions and model a story about the individual in the pictures. The children can then relay the story to uninformed listeners with the pictures removed. The adults can gradually lengthen the stories by adding more pictures and actions and by asking questions that will enable children to elaborate on the original story. In this way, more elaborate narrative structure will be elicited by modeling, elaboration, and expansion.

Specific Intervention Procedures for Narrative Content (NAP)

The six narrative dimensions may be targeted separately or together. For example, clinicians may find it more effective to focus on topic maintenance and event sequencing at the same time rather than separately. The rationale is that impairments of these dimensions frequently co-occur and it may well be more efficient to focus on two dimensions simultaneously. However, some children cannot attend to more than one dimension at a time and thus will need to devote separate attention to each.

Two other options are possible when working on NAP dimensions. Each dimension can be highlighted in different discourse genres before a second dimension is elicited. For example, professionals may focus on topic maintenance initially within scripts, then procedural discourse, and finally narratives. The same order could be used for event sequencing and informativeness.

An alternative approach would be to focus on each of the six dimensions within one genre before moving on to doing the six with another genre. In other words, the goal would be to improve all dimensions in scripts, followed by all dimensions in procedural discourse, and then narratives.

Which is more effective? Unfortunately, guidelines are not yet available to answer this question. Clinicians need to observe their clients and determine which approach will be most beneficial for them.

Topic Maintenance

1. Some children need to increase their auditory comprehension or attention because topic maintenance violations can result from an inability to understand or attend to what a conversational partner has said. In such instances, activities that are designed to increase children's ability to comprehend and pay attention should be implemented.
2. Contingent queries and verbal direction help a child to return to the original topic. The adult asks the child a question that serves to clarify a child's discourse or to return to the original topic.
3. Topic maintenance is achieved more easily in scripts and procedural discourse because they are more structured than personal narratives. These genres should be the starting points in therapy for children with severe narrative deficits.

Event Sequencing

1. Temporal words, such as *first, then,* and *last,* can function as anchor points. They may enable children to organize their thoughts.
2. For children with narrative difficulties, accurate event sequencing tends to decrease with added length and complexity. Therefore, simple and short passages should be attempted before longer and more complex forms. Also, events that occurred more recently or within a shorter time span may be easier to describe than those that occurred after a longer time span (Norris & Hoffman, 1993).
3. Describing events that have previously occurred highlight event sequencing. A child can enact an event, such as going to a doctor, and then describe the event to someone who was not present.

Informativeness

1. A task that enables a speaker to give directions or instructions to a naïve listener highlights the need to be informative. While this task does not constitute narrative, it may be used initially to emphasize the need to provide the listener with sufficient information. Narratives can be attempted after these skills have been achieved.

2. An adult can give an incomplete story and have the child ask contingent queries to obtain further information. The adult may need to model contingent queries initially. This procedure is useful to demonstrate that missing information creates a listener burden; that is, the listener does not understand what the speaker is trying to convey.

Children can be encouraged to provide more evaluation when an adult asks specific questions that will stimulate thinking about internal states, predictions, and inferences. For example, the following types of questions can be posed: "What did she feel?" "How were they going to do that?" "Why did it happen?" and "What will happen next?" Narratives should include evaluation because evaluation makes a narrative interesting and dynamic. Many speakers with language impairments do not provide an evaluative component, as was the case with some of the narratives in this book. Without evaluation, a speaker may give the impression of being impersonal and cold.

Referencing

Length of discourse and the narrator's social class are factors in referencing. As oral messages increase in length, children with language impairment struggle to provide adequate referencing (Purcell & Liles, 1992). Clinicians need to consider, however, that individuals from lower socioeconomic backgrounds who have no language impairment nonetheless habitually tend to use pronouns without previous identification (Hemphill, 1989). These factors need to be considered before targeting referencing for intervention.

1. To elicit appropriate referencing, professionals may want to use wordless picture books. An adult tells a story using a book that has many recurring characters so that adequate identification of pronouns is essential. The child then retells the story to an unfamiliar listener. The book must be removed in order to avoid reliance on visual aids or degeneration into picture description rather than narration.

2. Referencing in personal narratives should be targeted after fictional narratives (e.g., story retelling) have been used. The rationale for this procedure is that composing personal narratives is less structured than retelling fictional stories and presents additional challenges in terms of referencing. Clinicians need to ensure that the child can transfer skills from fictional to personal narrative.

3. Contingent queries during personal narration, as we have stressed, are useful as a means of signaling to the client that a referent was not clear.
4. Referencing by means of lexical specificity can be accomplished by increasing word retrieval abilities (German, 1992). Teaching vocabulary and facilitating word recall and retrieval are useful procedures (McGregor & Leonard, 1989).

Conjunctive Cohesion

Conjunctions should not receive considerable attention. Children with typical and impaired language development use them appropriately in most contexts, as we have seen, although even children without language impairment tend to over-rely on *and* and *and then* (Peterson & McCabe, 1987).

1. Appropriate use of a conjunction requires that a child understand its meaning. For example, forms that reflect causality and temporal relations need to be comprehended before a child is expected to use them meaningfully. Children typically link their utterances with *and* and *and then*; these forms do not generally need to be elicited, especially if the child is able to produce narratives.
2. Meaningful contexts need to be developed in which a conjunction is necessary (Bliss, 1993). For example, a clinician can model a story that has many temporal connectors other than *and then* (e.g., *next, last, when,* etc.). The child can then be asked to relay the same or a similar story that is based on sequencing events. Stories that involve causality can be modeled for a child. Then fictional and real stories that involve this concept can be elicited.

Fluency

1. Dysfluencies may signal an inability to plan discourse. If this is so, a speaker needs to be encouraged to plan a discourse before it is transmitted. The child can learn to organize and frame a narrative with specific components, such as settings, actions, participants, and evaluations.
2. Dysfluencies may also signal a word retrieval deficit. Children will need to have their vocabulary enriched and to use word retrieval strategies (German, 1992; McGregor & Leonard, 1989).

Implementation of Narrative Intervention Strategies

An example of narrative intervention will be shown with one child with SLI who produced a narrative in Chapter 3 (pp. 41, 122). The clinician asked him about a hospital visit. He used inappropriate discourse with respect to topic maintenance, event sequencing, informativeness, and fluency. He had variable abilities with respect to referencing and conjunctive cohesion. The aim of an intervention program for him is to improve the first three NAP dimensions because these are most critical in terms of discourse coherence. The other three pertain to more specific aspects of discourse and can be treated later. The following procedures would be undertaken:

D = Discourse Attempt
The adult elicits a narrative from the child.

I = Identification

The clinician segments the narrative into three components: before the speaker went to the hospital, events in the hospital, and what happened after he left the hospital. This analysis will help the boy focus on brief amounts of information in short passages. Each section should be worked on separately. For the first section, the adult would ask the child questions such as "Where did it happen? What was the first thing that happened? Then what happened? What happened after that?" In this step, the clinician discovers pertinent information regarding the child's experience.

M = Model

The clinician would model the first section of the narrative:
I was on the street. I was on my bike and going fast. I fell off my bike. I hurt myself because I fell off my bike.

E = Elicited production

The clinician would then ask the child to tell this part of the story or would coconstruct it with him by giving him the first part (e.g., I was on the street) and then asking him to finish the narrative (e.g., Then what happened?).

The clinician should then focus on the second and, after that, the final part of the narrative, using the same procedures as described above. The child should proceed to tell the narrative completely to an uninformed listener. Finally, the child should tell a new narrative about a similar experience. The new narrative can be divided into three parts, such as before, during, and after an event.

Programming for Classrooms

In preschools, narratives are important because of their positive relationship to literacy (see Chapter 2, for review of relevant research). Children need to be encouraged to present well-developed and coherent narratives before they attend school.

Some activities that elicit and foster narration in a preschool context are sharing time, description of field trip activities, and dramatic play. (Note that show-and-tell might seem to call for narratives, but often becomes more a description of objects displayed.)

Many teachers will want to foster narrative development. Specifically, teachers can (1) encourage children to elaborate their narratives, (2) appreciate children's narratives by commenting on their communicative attempts, (3) avoid interrupting children, and (4) model well-developed narratives themselves and/or bring in professional storytellers. Children can construct stories about historical events, interesting experiences on a field trip (avoid reiterating the itinerary), and dramatic personal experiences. Children also should be encouraged to develop stories in the context of dramatic play, where teachers can stimulate variation by systematically introducing new evocative prompts (e.g., for restaurant play, shoe store play, doctor's office scenarios, pretend school).

Parent Programs

Parent interventions are more successful than school-based intervention programs in enhancing narrative abilities in young children (Peterson, Jesso, & McCabe, 1999). One reason is that parents spend much more time with their children than do educators or clinicians, and much time and interaction is necessary to truly improve narrative ability. Personal narrative conversations form an integral part of the relationships between parents and children, so parents are natural collaborators for teachers and clinicians. However, some parents need to be trained to elicit and foster narrative abilities in the home (Peterson, Jesso, & McCabe, 1999). In the Appendix of this volume, we give the details of one such program. This successful parent program was designed to enhance the narrative abilities of preschool children from lower-class backgrounds (Peterson, Jesso, & McCabe, 1999). Parents were taught to elicit narratives by asking leading questions, listening, and following a child's conversational lead. They were taught the following skills to augment narrative abilities:

1. Elicit narratives at mealtime, bedtime, waiting in a doctor's office, and during car rides.
2. Model narratives about their own past experiences.
3. Use clarification requests and expansions to enable their child to elaborate narratives.

Meetings and phone calls were used to encourage parents to maintain the narrative enhancement strategies that they had learned. The results of this program revealed that the parents were able to improve the narrative abilities of their children, with the unforeseen side benefit that they also significantly increased their children's vocabulary.

In summary, intervention for narrative discourse is comprised of many steps. Initially, appropriate basic narration is targeted, followed by the improvement of the six dimensions of NAP. The DIME procedure is effective in increasing narrative coherence. Parents and teachers need to be included in intervention programming.

Part 3

Typical and Disordered Adult Narration in Various Cultures

9

General Overview of Typical and Impaired Adult Narration

Examples of Nonimpaired Narrative Discourse from Adult Speakers from Four Cultures

Oral narrative from 44-year-old European North American woman (from our files)

One day I went shopping to S____, and we have two cars—a black car and a white car. And I'm really terrible when I park in the parking lot. I have a habit of not really watching where I park. And this was around the holidays, so I parked my car. I run in. I'm doing all my shopping, running out. Time to leave the shopping center, and I'm getting in the parking lot and it's like, "Where did I park my car?" I can't remember where I parked my car. And I'm thinking, "Okay, I always drive the white car, so I have the white car. I think I know in what general area." (And this probably isn't about being lost, but I lost my car.) So here I am walking up and down the aisles looking for a white car, and I have all of these people who think I'm going to be jumping in my car and they will get my spot. Only I can't find my car. I was really embarrassed. So, after ten minutes of walking up and down, it dawns on me that I don't have the white car. I have the black car!

Some key points about her narrative are:

- Topic maintenance, event sequencing, informativeness, referencing, conjunctive cohesion, and fluency are unimpaired and typical of a woman from her background.
- She uses the historical present ("I run in. I'm doing all my shopping") to give a heightened sense of involvement to listeners—we are put in her shoes.
- She gives us an efficient narrative in the form valued by her culture. She begins with orientation as to where she went shopping and the cars she owns, proceeds to add to this evaluative description of herself as a poor parker of

cars, and then describes a series of events that constitute her search for her car. She marks the high point clearly ("Only I can't find my car. I was really embarrassed.") and resolves the narrative with the last two sentences. (See Chapter 3 for more detail regarding typical European North American narration.)

Oral narrative from 38-year-old Japanese bilingual man told in English (from Yoshimi Maeno, 2000)

Interviewer: Tell me about one time when you were injured.

Man: My injury story, story was when I was a 10 years old when I played soccer football. I, I slid to on the stone, and I I had cut my head. And th, uhh, I didn't, didn't know what happened. But, uhhh, some teammate asked me what happened on your head. And I had a lot of blood of, on my face. And some, uh, students called a ambulance and, uh, I I was took to the hospital. And, uh, the doctor said to me oh I needed to stay at the hospital at least for two weeks. But uhh, I didn't feel so much big problem. I enjoyed the even the staying in that uh, uhh, at the hospital like a just like a hotel. So I, I walking around. Walked around uh hospital to have to look into, look for something interesting, so Doctor said to me, "You need to go away." (Laugh). Just in a one week. (Laugh).

Some key aspects of this narrative include:

- The narrator is concise, as is valued in Japanese culture.
- This story pertains to one experience, more typical of English than Japanese narration. The narrator has, perhaps incidentally, adopted the discourse style characteristic of the United States (See Chapter 6 for more detail regarding Asian and Asian American narration.)
- A few awkward phrases ("I was took to the hospital," "But I didn't feel so much big problem," "So I walking around") and some deletions (omitted subject in "Walked around hospital") may be importations from Japanese.
- Note the presence of a number of dysfluencies, which can be quite typical of individuals for whom English is a second language (e.g., repetitions of *I*).

Oral narrative from 42-year-old Mexican American man (from our files)

Interviewer: I saw a car broken down on my way here. Have you ever been in a car accident?

Client: It happen to me!

Interviewer: What happen to you? Tell me.

Client: Accident. I crashed into a post. That is it!

Interviewer: Oh, what else? What else? How did it happen?

Client: And another car too. Ah.

Interviewer: Oh.

Client: And it ended in pie . . . ces.

Interviewer: I am sorry. I did not hear you.

Client: Into pieces.

Interviewer: Wow, what happen next?

Client: I was a month in a coma.

Interviewer: Oh wow, and after that?

Client: After, I came to here.

Key points include:

- The succinctness of the preceding example might partly be due to the fact that the interviewer did not truly maintain this as a conversation, a feature of Spanish narration. (See Chapter 5 for more detail regarding Spanish and Spanish American narration.) At the time of the interview, this man reported feeling uncomfortable with the neutral prompts delivered by the interviewer. He was looking for personal narratives from her that would have been more personable and engaging—a true attempt to forge a bond. In the absence of this, the speaker chose not to elaborate what he said.
- Spanish word order is imported into this English narrative (e.g., "I was a month in a coma").
- The speaker displays limited fluency in his second language, English, yet tells the full gist of his experience. (See Chapter 5 for more detail regarding typical Spanish-English narration.)

Oral narrative from 47-year-old African American woman (from our files)
Interviewer: Have you ever been in a car accident?

Woman: Yes I have. It was the year of 1980. Uh, I was coming to work. I had gone to, uh, drop a friend off that was riding with me. On the way back, it was on Thanksgiving day in November. It was raining and a car came off the freeway onto the feeder road at the speed of 55 miles per hour. Apparently, there was something wrong with the light because the light wouldn't turn from I think it was like red and then yellow and then green and then back to red again. Uh, this Oldsmobile, it had to been like a 1965 model. My car was a brand new Corvette made of fiberglass. It ended up being a mess. There was glass everywhere and my head hit the windshield. I was about three months pregnant and when the police came, he asked me what happened. At the time I could not begin to even put together what took place. Uh, I gave him a few minutes. He went . . . He knew I couldn't tell him what happened. He went to the next couple and they gave him their side of the story. After that, I uh had someone call my family and we went to the emergency room and they had to take glass out of my forehead. Uh, it injured the side of my stomach, but the baby wasn't hurt. And uh that was it. I had my car only two months and had to invest in a new car. That happened in 1980 and then the insurance paid it off and then I got another new car.

Some key points include:

- This narrative is the kind of classic personal narrative that is favored by African and European North Americans. It begins with orientation (exact year, background activity, that it happened on Thanksgiving), goes through a series of actions that culminate in the high point, the car crash, which is heavily evaluated ("It ended up being a mess . . . He went . . . ").

- Listeners may be puzzled that the narrator did not explicitly restate the actual event of the car crash itself (which can be easily inferred from her assent to the interviewer's prompt). However, this omission of the traumatic event is both typical (there is a long history in psychology of amnesia for trauma) and accounted for in this particular narrative ("He knew I couldn't tell him what happened").
- The narrator resolves the narrative by explaining that she called her family and went to the hospital and settled with the insurance company.
- This narrative pertains to one topic—one experience, actually, despite the fact that at times some African Americans prefer to tell a narrative that combines several thematically related experiences (see Chapter 4 for more detail regarding African American narration).
- Event sequencing is not a focus of this story, but neither is it violated.
- There is quite a bit of specific information, elaboration, and inclusion of action, description, and evaluation here. The only aspect of informativeness in question has been dealt with above (i.e., specification of actual traumatic event).
- Referencing is explicit for the most part, which is typical of middle-class individuals. The few references that are not specific ("they had to take glass out of my forehead") are acceptable colloquial references to authority figures.
- Conjunctions are interesting to consider in this example. This narrator does not rely upon *and* heavily, though there are several instances of its use. She also uses *and when*, and *but*. However, the most interesting point is that she has substituted much more sophisticated and specific conjunctive devices for the common conjunctions; she uses connectives such as *On the way back, Apparently, At the time, After that*.
- Dysfluencies include only rare filled pauses.
- In spite of the trauma of the experience, this speaker has made a coherent story of it afterwards. She has literally gotten her story together.

Adults' versus Children's Narratives from Different Cultural Backgrounds

Systematic comparison of the personal narratives of adults from different cultures has recently received some attention, and cultural differences have been documented. Carmella Peréz (1998) compared personal narratives from Puerto Rican adults to those of European North Americans and found a number of differences: (1) English narratives had a significantly longer pause at the outset of narration, indicative of up-front planning, while Spanish narratives had a significantly greater percentage of false starts and corrections and within-narrative pauses and silences—reflective of planning while narrating. (2) Spanish narratives had a greater percentage of referential cohesion than did English narratives. (3) Spanish narratives contained significantly fewer formal openings and closings than did English narratives. (4) While the classic narrative structure was the most common structure of the personal narratives of English speakers, Spanish speakers told narratives of multiple experiences just as often as they did classic narratives of a single experience. There were no cultural differences in productivity, however.

Similarly, Yoshimi Maeno (2000) compared adult narratives in Japanese and English from native Japanese- and native English-speaking bilingual adults. Specifically, she found the following differences, among others: (1) Japanese narration consisted of more turns than did English narration. (2) Statements in Japanese narrative were shorter than in English. (3) Japanese narration tends to consist of three-line stanzas (see Chapter 1), whereas English narration consists of collections of anywhere between one and six lines. (4) Japanese narration uses the past progressive ("Were talking") more so than English, which tends to consist of sequences of simple past-tense events. (5) Japanese narration combines several distinct experiences, whereas English narration elaborates upon one such experience. (6) Japanese narration uses relatively more orientation, while English narration uses relatively more evaluation. (7) Japanese narration often uses subject and object ellipsis, while English narration does not.

In other words, listeners find systematic cultural differences in adult narration when they carefully examine productions. Nonetheless, when we consider the examples at the outset of this chapter, we would have to say that differences among adults from different cultures seem more muted than those among children. We speculate that this is due, perhaps, to the homogenizing effects of schooling and/or to these adults' increased exposure to a variety of discourse styles. As with children, clinicians and educators working with adults from different cultural backgrounds are advised to keep an open mind about whether cultural differences are operating.

Standard Tests versus Narrative Assessment

As with children, the narrative ability of adults needs to be assessed independently of their performance on other aspects of language such as those in typical aphasia batteries. For example, intact use of all six narrative dimensions is present in the following narrative from a stroke victim. We might expect impairments in discourse coherence as a result of her stroke. We might also expect some features of African American discourse (described in Chapter 4). However, none of these features is present.

> ***Oral narrative of a 49-year-old African American woman with right hemispheric stroke (from our files):***
> **Examiner:** My neighbor had his car stolen last night. He went outside and it was gone. He was really mad. Have you ever had something stolen? Tell me about it.
>
> **Client:** (1) I was home . . . (2) I was home . . . (3) and this is holiday coming up holiday . . . Christmas (4) And I'm a fool. (5) I go to the bank. (6) And I get $1500.

... (7) and put it in this big old pocketbook ... (8) sit it beside me. (9) And, little did I know...those boys was watching me when I got out of the car. (10) I never did lock my door.... (11) When I got out of my car, they took my whole pocketbook, money and all, keys to the house and everything.... (12) That was a weird-ass feeling.... (13) Then I went to see the parents 'cause I knew them. (14) And the parents cussed me out ... (15) told me to get the hell away from them.

In this narrative the six dimensions of narrative discourse are appropriately used:

Topic Maintenance: Appropriate. The speaker describes only the events relating to the theft of her purse.

Event Sequencing: Appropriate. The speaker describes the events in chronological order.

Informativeness: Appropriate. There is sufficient information for the listener to be able to understand the narrative. The story is elaborated; description (utterances 2, 3), action (utterances 5, 6, 7, etc.) and evaluation (utterances 4, 7, 9, 12, etc.) are present.

Referencing: Appropriate. The listener easily understands the references. For example, in utterance 7, the expression " ... this big old pocketbook" is colloquial usage. Reference to "the parents" (utterance 13) is clear from the context. The speaker is able to identify specific referents, such as home, holiday, and bank. She uses pronouns with prior antecedents (utterances 8, 12, and 13).

Conjunctive Cohesion: Appropriate. The speaker uses conjunctions for semantic purposes, such as coordination (utterances 3, 4, 6, etc.) and temporal (utterance 13), and causal (utterance 13) semantic purposes, as well as for pragmatic purposes (utterance 9—change of focus).

Fluency: Appropriate. The few dysfluencies that occur do not disrupt discourse coherence (the repetitions in utterances 1, 2, and 3 may be a discourse strategy designed to emphasize a point). While some individuals with right brain damage have reduced discourse coherence (Glosser, 1993), this speaker does not show such impairments. Her narrative is coherent, complete, and easily understood. Moreover, this speaker shows a strong use of evaluation that makes her narrative vibrant.

Overview of Adult Impairments in the Six Dimensions of NAP

Previous research regarding the narrative discourse of adults with impairments has focused on a limited set of parameters, such as cohesion (Ripich & Terrel, 1988; Simmons-Mackie & Damico, 1996;), referencing (Nicholas & Brookshire, 1993; Nicholas, Obler, Albert, & Helm-Estabrooks, 1985), topic maintenance (Glosser & Deser, 1990;

Glosser, 1993; Mentis & Prutting, 1991; Mentis, Briggs, & Gramigna, 1995), or story grammar (Roman, Brownell, Potter, Siebold, & Gardner, 1987; Ska & Guenard, 1993). These aspects of discourse coherence are generally viewed independently of each other, which does not offer professionals the opportunity to determine which of many possible dimensions should be targeted in intervention. In the NAP a broader set of relevant discourse dimensions are considered simultaneously in order to provide a more comprehensive assessment of discourse coherence. Note that for readers of prior chapters on children, some of this information about adults will be redundant. We have included such redundant information here for readers who are focused on adults.

Topic Maintenance

This dimension focuses on the extent to which utterances are related to a given topic. Off-topic discourse patterns consist of inclusion of extraneous, tangential, or associative information. Discourse coherence will be disrupted if the listener cannot follow the topic of conversation. Confusion will result because the listener does not know what topic to focus on.

Topic maintenance disorders are characteristic of a variety of adult communicative impairments. For example, violations in topic maintenance have been reported for individuals with dementia of the Alzheimer's type (DAT) (Bayles, Kasniak, & Tomoeda, 1987; Chenery & Canter, 1990; Grafman, Thompson, Weingartner, Martinez, Lawlor, & Sunderland, 1991; Mentis, Briggs, & Gramigna, 1995; Nicholas, Olber, Albert, & Helm-Estabrooks, 1985). Symptoms include tangential and irrelevant utterances as well as narrative paraphasias in which irrelevant mininarrative segments are incorporated in a speaker's original narrative (Cardebat, Demonet, & Doyon, 1993). In contrast, adults with right brain damage and traumatic brain injury have variable topic maintenance disorders (George & Johnson, 1995; Glosser & Deser, 1990; Frederiksen & Stemmer, 1993; Mentis & Prutting, 1991; McDonald, 1992; Myers, 1993). Some adults with right brain injury and traumatic brain injury may show adequate topic maintenance (Bloom, Borod, Obler, & Gerstman, 1993; Glosser, 1993; Prutting & Kirchner, 1987).

Event Sequencing

The presentation of events in chronological order constitutes another dimension of narration. Unless a speaker indicates that an intentional violation of ordering will occur, events should be presented in chronological sequence in most cultures. When events are not presented chronologically, listeners may have difficulty following the order of events.

Event sequencing problems have been reported in the discourse of adults with right brain damage (Myers, 1993) and dementia of the Alzheimer's type (DAT) (Grafman et al., 1991; Ska & Guenard, 1993). Impairments have been characterized by achronological sequencing in spontaneous discourse, scripts, and fictional stories. Intact event sequencing appears to be generally intact in the procedural discourse of adults with aphasia, however (Ulatowska et al., 1983).

Informativeness

This dimension of narrative discourse refers to the sense-making aspect of discourse coherence and includes issues of completeness and elaboration. When a narrative is incomplete or unelaborated, a listener will have difficulty in understanding it. There are three specific aspects of narrative informativeness that are analogous to the different requirements of a police officer, a teacher, and a cook.

When a police officer asks a witness to give an account of what happened during an accident or crime, she or he asks for "just the facts." Basic information about an experience needs to be presented in a narrative in order for it to be coherent and useful. This first aspect relates to whether the information that is presented is sufficient for listeners to make sense of the narrative.

These basic facts are not always enough, however. That is, a teacher often will ask a student to elaborate on narratives at school. The elaborated version would provide the listener with a more complete understanding of the speaker's message. This second aspect refers to how well narratives are generally elaborated. Optional details help make a text engaging. However, some speakers are taciturn or reticent to elaborate narrative detail. They will only provide the gist of a description.

Narrators may present enough facts to please a police officer or even elaborate on the facts enough for a teacher and still leave listeners dissatisfied, like a cook who omits critical spices from some dish. Thus the third aspect of informativeness consists of basic components that should be present but may be systematically deleted from a narrative: specifically, description, action, and evaluation should all be present (Labov, 1972). Descriptions consist of attributions of people or objects, while actions are actual events. Evaluation relates the significance of an event for a speaker (Labov, 1972). Adjectives, descriptions of internal states, exclamations, and negatives are some of the common types of evaluations encountered in personal narratives. A complete list of evaluations can be found in Chapter 1 (Labov, 1972; McCabe & Rollins, 1994; Peterson & McCabe, 1983). Evaluation may seem to represent an optional aspect of narration because it does not have a significant impact on a plot and consists of some relatively complex syntactic devices (i.e., comparatives, modals, and negatives) (Labov, 1972; Ulatowska et al., 1981). However, it is prominent in the narratives of many African American (Labov, 1972), European North American (Peterson & McCabe, 1983), Puerto Rican (Peréz, 1998), and Japanese (Minami, 1996) adults. If evaluation is missing, the narrative may make adequate sense but will not be universally satisfying.

Reductions in informativeness are characteristic of a variety of adult communicative disorders. Incomplete narratives and discourse have been reported for adults with right brain injury (George & Johnson, 1995; Hough, 1990; Moya, Benowitz, Levine, & Finkelstein, 1986; Roman, Brownell, Potter, Siebold, & Gardner, 1987; Sherratt & Penn, 1990; Wapner, Hamby, & Gardner, 1981; Weylman, Brownell, Roman, & Gardner, 1989), adults with dementia of the Alzheimer's type (Cardebat, Demonet, & Doyon, 1993; Chenery & Canter, 1990; Chenery & Murdock, 1994; Mentis et al., 1995; Ripich & Terrel, 1988; Ska & Guenard, 1993), and adults with traumatic brain injury (Glosser & Deser, 1990; Hartley & Jensen, 1991, 1992; Liles, Coelho, Duffy, & Zalagens, 1989; Mentis & Prutting, 1991). The characteristics across these disorders are reduced informational content, omitted narrative components, decreased detail and elaboration, inaccurate information, and implicitness. Evaluation may be absent because a speaker is unable to use complex language or does not realize the importance of this component in discourse (Ulatowska et al., 1981).

Referencing

This dimension represents the identification of individuals, features, and events (Halliday & Hassan, 1976). Referencing varies according to the ethnicity and socio-economic background of a speaker. For example, African American speakers do not always completely identify persons or locations (Michaels, 1981, 1991). They rely on the listener to fill in aspects of the discourse. Similarly, European North American speakers from low-income backgrounds do not always specify their referents (Hemphill, 1989). In such communities, the listener habitually serves as a discourse collaborator who fills in unstated information (Hemphill, 1989).

For impaired European North American speakers who come from middle class backgrounds, four types of referencing errors may occur (Glosser, Wiener, & Kaplan, 1988): (1) Inadequate articles or proper noun references may be evident. This type of error is characterized by the substitution of a definite for an indefinite article (*the* for *a*) or the use of names of people and places without prior identification. (2) Indefinite noun references, such as *this*, *thing*, or *people*, may be used in place of specific words. (3) Confused pronoun references occur when agreement between a pronoun and its referent does not occur. An example is "Jane was so mad that *he* left early." (4) Omitted or misrepresented references are characterized by deleted or inaccurate references as in the utterance "gave me gift," in which the agent has not been specified. Neologisms and paraphasias would also be placed in this category.

Referencing is a major area of difficulty for adults with a variety of communicative disorders. Adults with Wernicke's aphasia and DAT have serious referencing problems. For example, both disorders are characterized by empty speech consisting of indefinite noun references (Cardebat, Demonet, & Doyon, 1993; Chenery & Murdock, 1994; Mentis et al., 1995; Nicholas et al., 1985; Ulatowska et al., 1988). Demonstrative pronouns, such as *this*, *there*, and *that*, are used without prior identification and reflect indefinite noun references (Nicholas et al., 1985). Pronouns without antecedents reduce discourse coherence (Nicholas et al., 1985). Adults with Wernicke's aphasia have their discourse coherence further reduced by literal and verbal paraphasias and neologisms in comparison to individuals with DAT (Nicholas et al., 1985). In contrast, referencing will be variable in adults with right brain damage and traumatic brain injury (Bloom et al., 1993; Glosser, 1993; Glosser & Deser, 1990; McDonald, 1992; Mentis & Prutting, 1991; Tompkins, 1995; Prutting & Kirchner, 1987).

Conjunctive Cohesion

Conjunctive cohesion refers to the words that link utterances, words such as *and, but, so*. Utterances may be joined either semantically or pragmatically using these conjunctions. Without appropriate links, a text will be disjointed and a little difficult for a listener to comprehend.

Two types of cohesion are evident in discourse. Semantic connectives link utterances according to their meaning (Liles, 1985; Peterson & McCabe, 1991). For example, coordination represents the description of a series of events that are not temporally ordered. Temporal links connect segments with respect to chronological ordering. Causal relationships may be expressed, as well as disjuncture, in which utterances or phrases are contrasted. Enabling relations describe precausal relationships between utterances and are frequently denoted by use of *so*.

Conjunctive cohesion may also be evident as pragmatic links between utterances (Peterson & McCabe, 1991). Connectives can serve to begin or end discourse segments. They can also signal changes in a predicted chronological or sequential ordering of events. Adults with nonfluent aphasia have been shown to use discourse markers in order to regulate and maintain discourse (Simmons-Mackie & Damico, 1996).

Disruptions in conjunctive cohesion are variable in many adult communication disorders. Breakdowns are not an identifying characteristic in the discourse of individuals with traumatic brain injury (Liles et al., 1989). In DAT the results are mixed. Nicholas and colleagues (1985) reported the use of nonmeaningful conjunctions, while other researchers have found relatively intact use of conjunctions (Glosser & Deser, 1990; Ripich & Terrell, 1988). Adult aphasia may be characterized by an increase in errors and/or a restricted range of conjunctions (Ulatowska & Bond, 1983; Ulatowska, North, & Malcaluso-Haynes, 1981). However, caution needs to be exercised in considering errors of conjunctive cohesion because previously only semantic analyses were conducted on these forms. A form that might have been considered to reflect a semantic misusage may reflect a discourse function. For example, Ulatowska and colleagues (1981) gave the following utterance as an example of an error in conjunctive use: "She will be 46 on her birthday *but* we lived out in the country and had to have a man to come out there (p. 361)." This usage could be considered to represent the pragmatic function of change of focus in the discourse. In short, a broader analysis of conjunctions, including pragmatic as well as semantic usage, might reflect additional strengths in conjunctive cohesion for adults with communicative disorders.

Fluency

Fluency refers to the manner of production of narrative. Three types of dysfluencies may be identified: (1) False starts are abandoned utterances. (2) Internal corrections consist of retracings of words and phrases. (3) Repetitions are redundant and nonevaluative reiterations of lexical items. Hesitations, pauses, and fillers also disrupt the manner of production, but do not reduce discourse coherence and therefore are not considered here.

Dysfluencies are characteristic of various types of aphasia. For example, Broca's aphasia—also termed "nonfluent" aphasia—is characterized by short bursts of speech. Pauses, internal corrections, fillers, and false starts are evident. All types of aphasia are characterized by dysfluencies, some of which may be related to word retrieval deficits. The discourse of adults with DAT and traumatic brain injury is also characterized by dysfluencies (Biddle, McCabe, & Bliss, 1996; Hartley & Jensen, 1991, 1992; Marsh & Knight, 1991; McDonald, 1993; Ripich & Terrell, 1988). Individuals with the former disorder may have incomplete utterances while those with the latter disorder will show hesitations, fillers, repetitions, and false starts.

10

Examples of Impaired Adult Narrative Discourse

In this section we will present the narratives of adults in order to show the range of discourse impairments that can be described within the framework of the NAP (see Table 10.1, page 150). This assessment procedure was not designed to make differential diagnoses among impairments—there are too many overlapping symptoms for that to be a reasonable objective. However, the NAP enables us to develop profiles of impairments, both for groups in general (see group profile of adults and children with traumatic brain injury in Biddle et al., 1996) and, as is our purpose in this chapter, for individuals.

> *Example from 75-year-old, European North American middle-class man with mild nonfluent (Broca's) aphasia (from our files)*
> **Interviewer:** Did you ever have anything stolen?
>
> **Client:** (1) Yeah, it was stuff that were "blob" in to get my uh people that were gettin' out . . . excuse me . . . stuff that they . . . these . . . they tried to get out of the house. (2) And took some of our good stuff, our jeweleries, before even the fre . . . meec . . . got there (3) But we never didn't see it. (4) They also broke along the side of the heart into the house in order to get out.

Topic Maintenance: Appropriate. All the utterances relate to one topic.

Event Sequencing: Appropriate. The events are presented chronologically.

Informativeness: Variable. The narrative is generally explicit. There is enough information for the listener to understand the gist of the experience. However, the narrative is not elaborated. This terse style may reflect the Broca's aphasia and/or a taciturn nature. Some action (utterances 1, 2, and 4) and evaluation (utterances 2 and 3) are present. However, description is nonexistent.

Referencing: Variable. Most problems encountered concern referencing. One area of deficit is with the use of indefinite noun references, such as the use of

149

TABLE 10.1 *Narrative Assessment Profile*

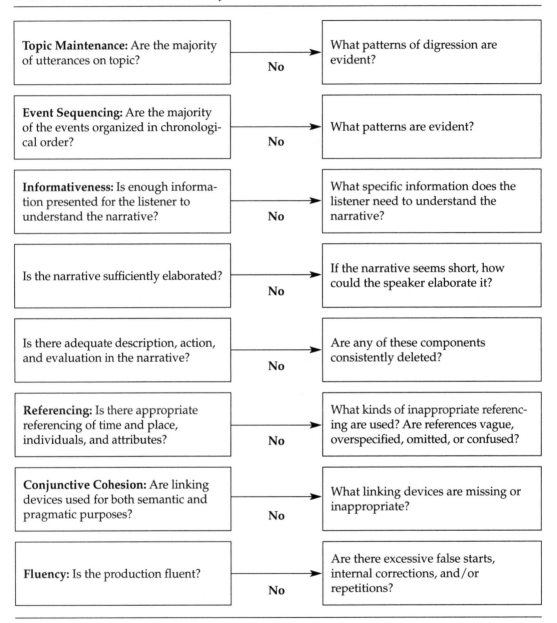

"people" and "stuff" (utterance 1). The speaker also has omitted or misrepresented references. He uses a neologism (utterance 1, "blob") and a literal paraphasia (utterance 2, "fre . . . meec"), which is a phonetic form that appears to be related to the target, *police*. The use of pronouns is not always specified (utterances 1, 2, 3, and 4); however, we can guess their meanings from the context of the narrative. More specification would increase the coherence of the narrative.

Conjunctive Cohesion: Appropriate. The speaker uses two conjunctions, one for a semantic (utterance 2, coordination) and one for a pragmatic (utterance 3, change of focus) purpose. A longer text may have resulted in additional conjunctions.

Fluency: Variable. While there is some fluent speech, there are also internal corrections (utterances 1 and 2).

Intervention Goals. Intervention should initially focus on elaboration of discourse. The speaker needs to include more descriptions and evaluation in his narrative discourse. Referencing, in the form of word retrieval, should also be an area of focus.

> *Example from 44-year-old African American man with Broca's (nonfluent) aphasia (from our files)*
> **Interviewer:** Have you ever been in a car accident?
>
> **Client:** (1) Uh, not like that.
>
> **Interviewer:** No?
>
> **Client:** (2) Uh-huh. I think I've been in one where uh just this, it hit the front side of both of us, you know. (3) We just slid just a little bit. (4) There was really no damage.
>
> **Interviewer:** Uh-huh. Tell me more.
>
> **Client:** (5) Well that was it.
>
> **Interviewer:** Then what happened.
>
> **Client:** (6) Well, uh, well he hit us. (7) And then we slid a little bit, (8) and we, uh, you know, that's just the way. (9) That's just. (10) Oh boy. (11) That's it. (12) That was the accident.

Topic Maintenance: Appropriate. All utterances refer to the accident.

Event Sequencing: Appropriate. The speaker presents the few events in plausible order.

Informativeness: Inappropriate. Although this speaker is from a culture that values length, this is a remarkable short narrative. One gets the distinct sense from the speaker's frustrated exclamation "Oh boy" at the end that he had more to tell, but simply could not. He includes action ("slid") and evaluation ("really no damage"), but no orientation to speak of.

Referencing: Needs further study. Most references are unspecified pronouns. Clinicians would want to determine from the speaker's family members just how much of a deficit it represents. Perhaps he always had an implicit, collaborative style, depending on listeners to flesh out information.

Conjunctive Cohesion: Appropriate. The speaker only used one *and then*, but this omission is minor compared to his other discourse impairment.

Fluency: Variable. While there are remarkably few repeated phrases, discontinued sentences, or corrected phrases, this speaker nonetheless seems dysfluent from the way that he seemed to bail out of the telling at the end.

Intervention Goals.   Increased informativeness and referencing are needed to improve this speaker's discourse coherence.

Example from 79-year-old African American woman with fluent (Wernicke's) aphasia (from our files)
In the following narrative, a woman describes an experience with a stolen car. She uses some African English Vernacular forms (e.g., utterances 9 and 18) and comes from a relatively low socioeconomic background, which is relevant to referencing practices.

Client: (1) I heard of it, yes.

Interviewer: Can you tell me about that?

Client: (2) Well, upstairs uh right here uh . . . girl stole my li, my uh car . . . up, up uh. . . . (3) And I go all around looking around. (4) I did find the woman that had caught my head (5) And and um she parked it away somewhere (6) and would would kept would with the police (7) and they find my re my red uh . . . (8) can't find my keys. (9) She done took my keys (10) But I can't . . . (11) but I got another pair (12) And I get my find (13) and she rep found that uh uh woman that caught my car (14) and she got time and take. . . . (15) They put her in jail. (16) I don't know (17) And uh my my daughter said where sitting before (18) And uh she seen a couple times back to that before she be put up about three months. . . . (19) So so I don't know. (20) But uh it happened to me. (21) But that's all of it.

Topic Maintenance: Appropriate. All events focus on the stolen car.

Event Sequencing: Appropriate. The speaker presents the events in chronological order.

Informativeness: Variable. The narrative is generally informative. There is sufficient elaboration of information for the listener to understand the message; major violations of sense making are not evident. Some descriptions are present (in utterance 7, the speaker mentions red but cannot provide the object, presumably her car; in utterance 2, the speaker may be trying to say "little" but cannot retrieve the complete word). In contrast, there is a lot of action (utterances 2, 3, 4, 5, etc.). This narrative is unusual, however, in its lack of evaluation. The only instance is one negative (utterance 8). As was mentioned earlier, evaluation is common in the narratives of speakers of African American descent (Labov, 1972). We can contrast this absence with the narrative about the 1980 car wreck on page 139, in which evaluation was abundant, giving the listener a clear idea of how the speaker felt and some indication of her personality. In this narrative about the stolen car, the listener does not get such information; the narrative seems bereft of any feeling.

Referencing: Variable. Strengths consist of adequate pronoun and noun references: *she* refers to the thief and her daughter (utterances 5, 9, 14, 18), *it* (utterance 5) refers to the car; and *they* refers to the police (utterances 7, 15). The speaker is also able to identify specific references, such as car (utterance 2), keys (utterances 8, 9), jail (utterance 15), and daughter (utterance 17) in spite of a dysnomia which is characteristic of fluent aphasia. However, there are instances of ambiguous referents as evidenced by semantic and verbal paraphasias. Some examples are evident in utterances 4 ("caught my head"; the first word is a semantic paraphasia and the last word, an unrelated verbal paraphasia), 12 ("find" is an unrelated verbal paraphasia), and 13 (in "caught my car" the first word is a semantic paraphasia). The phrases in utterance 18 ("couple of times back" and "put up") may represent colloquial or idiomatic speech or may be semantic paraphasias.

Conjunctive Cohesion: Appropriate. The speaker uses conjunctions for both semantic and pragmatic purposes. For example, the conjunctions *and* and *but* are used semantically for coordination (utterances 5, 6, 7, etc.) and disjuncture (utterance 11). The conjunctions *so* and *but* are used pragmatically for closure (utterances 19, 20, and 21).

Fluency: Inappropriate. Several types of dysfluencies are evident that reduce discourse coherence: false starts (utterances 7, 10, 14), and repetitions (utterances 2, 3, 5, 6, 7, 19).

Intervention Goals.   This speaker also has an uneven profile reflecting various strengths and weaknesses. Topic maintenance, event sequencing, most areas of informativeness, and conjunctive cohesion are appropriate while her narrative suffers from the lack of evaluation, variable referencing, and dysfluencies. Thus, informativeness and referencing are appropriate targets for this adult. The speaker needs to increase the identification of individuals as part of decreasing her dysnomia. Word retrieval deficits should receive focus because they reduce the coherence of all kinds of discourse, including narrative. Improvements in word retrieval may also increase fluency. The second aspect of narration that should receive focus is evaluation, which is expected for African American speakers (Labov, 1972). Its absence reduces the effectiveness of the narrative.

Example from African American woman with fluent (Wernicke's) aphasia
(left cardiovascular accident, from our files)

Interviewer: Have you ever bought a house?

Client: Yah, well I had the the the door was was was. I guess it was fixed up with the thing. The stuff in there withouth somebody seeing that and made it good for everbody. And I sosher . . . XXX and it sosher. That's all I can tell ya.

Interviewer: Tell me more.

Client: Well, it's its's a prettiest dress and you have a dirty clothes and everthing is clean right now. It's just for you.

Topic Maintenance: Needs further study. Pressed by the interviewer to expand her narrative, this patient seems to have switched topics. Perhaps the two topics are thematically related (see Chapter 4), and the clinician should be encouraged to ask her family and/or friends about whether they are. However, it seems likely that this narrator has difficulty with topic maintenance as defined by the African American community.

Event Sequencing: Needs further study. This cannot be determined because there are no recognizable events that could be sequenced.

Informativeness: Inappropriate. Because the African American community values lengthy narration, we can say that this narrative—especially if it were the lengthiest one she could produce—was deficient by the standards of her community. Intervention and/or understanding of this difficulty are called for. Neither event is given in sufficient detail to understand the gist, let alone elaborated. The narrative contains no actions nor much orientation.

Referencing: Inappropriate. The speaker does not provide adequate identification for words, such as "stuff," "thing," and "it." This person also uses "sosher," which represents a paraphasia.

Conjunctive Cohesion: Inappropriate. The speaker uses two *ands* to connect utterances that themselves are reduced in coherence.

Fluency: Variable. This short discourse has a few word repetitions and one false start. Most of the speaker's utterances are fluent, however.

Intervention Goals.   Informativeness and referencing are appropriate goals. The speaker should learn to provide more facts as well as evaluation in narration. References need to be specified appropriately.

Example from 73-year-old European North American woman with conduction
aphasia (from our files)

The speaker in the following narrative is middle class at present, although the construction "they done it" is typical of lower-class dialect.

Interviewer: Have you ever had anything stolen?

Client: (1) Right over here they did [steal something]. (2) And my husband was . . .
(3) He heard somebody walking out there. (4) And it was late at night . . . (5)

And he, he heard something bang bong, you know. (6) Now the people next door didn't hear it . . . (7) But . . . he he opened up the uh . . . (8) He said, "Where are you going? (9) What are you doing over there?"(10) And he took all the things out. (11) And he started running. (12) So my husband went with running, you know. (13) I said, "What are you doing to be with him?"(14) And there was two uh uh . . . rrrr, you know?

Interviewer: Two cars?

Client: (15) Yeah, the co-, no the ones's with the kinda pick 'em up, you know. (16) When they looking to check 'em. (17) And then he'd say, "I'm glad you found that man. (18) Because we went all over to look. (19) We'd been c- going all the h-houses. (20) And he was taking all the things he ruined." (21) And I was so glad I didn't get mine to be ruined too. (22) Yeah, a lot of them say that they done it.

Topic Maintenance: Appropriate. All the utterances relate to the theft the narrator experienced.

Event Sequencing: Appropriate. The events are presented in a plausible, probable sequence.

Informativeness: Variable. The narrative is fairly incoherent. It seems as if specific information about the experience is missing and hard to infer. For example, between utterances 7 and 8, we suspect that the husband saw the thief, though we should have been told that. However, the narrative is sufficiently long—simple elaboration is not the issue here. As far as the third aspect of informativeness is concerned, there is description (utterances 1, 4, 14, 15, 22), action (utterances 3, 5, 7, 8, 9, 10, 11, 12, 13, 16, 17, 18, 19, 20), and evaluation (utterances 6, 21).

Referencing: Variable. There is appropriate identification of the husband and the people next door. There are ambiguous references to location in utterances 1 ("right over here") and 3 ("there"), and to participants in utterances 1, 16, 17, 21, as well as in utterance 10 (where "he" changes from use to refer to husband to use to refer to thief, and utterance 21, among others).

This narrative contains numerous symptoms of aphasia that are not specific to narrative although they reduce narrative discourse coherence. There is a paraphasia in utterance 15 ("pick 'em up" for "pick-up truck"). Utterances 12 and 16 are so oddly phrased it is hard to classify the problem. Utterance 14 reflects a word-finding problem. The use of *ruined* in utterances 20 and 21 is a lexical substitution for *stole*.

Conjunctive Cohesion: Variable, mostly appropriate. *And* is used for coordination in utterances 2, 4, 5, etc. *So* is used causally to show the husband's motivation for running, if you assume that the "he" in the previous sentence referred to the thief. *But* is ambiguous because utterance 7 is incomplete. The use of *because* in utterance 18 seems a genuine error.

Fluency: Inappropriate. Speaker has numerous false starts (utterances 2, 7, 14), internal corrections (utterances 15, 19), and repetitions (utterances 5, 7).

Intervention Goals. Most global narrative abilities are intact for this individual. She has strengths in topic maintenance and event sequencing, as well as some in informativeness. Conjunctive cohesion is mostly intact. Priorities for intervention with this individual relate to informativeness, referencing, and fluency. She needs to provide more specific information for her listeners. Her fluency difficulties can be addressed by improving word-retrieval abilities.

The narrative of this speaker illustrates how complex the issue of narrative referencing can be in clinical settings. We suspect, as noted above, that she grew up in a lower class environment, so we would also expect her to use an ambiguous referencing style regardless of her current income. However, she has aphasia and her referencing is quite impaired. Thus, professionals might want to work on referencing from the standpoint of what the listener really needs to know (i.e., cannot easily infer from context).

Example from 93-year-old European North American with unspecified dementia (from our files)
The following narrative represents a severe disorder of discourse coherence. The speaker, from a middle-class background, has a dementia that has not been classified. She resides in a nursing home. She earned a score of 13.30 on the Mini-mental state examination (Folstein, Folstein, & McHugh, 1975), which indicates a moderately severe impairment.

Interviewer: Have you ever had anything stolen?

Client: (1) Actually I was very worried about what was taken from me . . . papers (2) And I'm a collector of stamps mostly. (3) They were most important. (4) They have been, shall we say, stole to people before.

Interviewer: What happened?

Client: (5) Well, I check when they came in here (6) And they kind of moved.

Interviewer: They moved?

Client: (7) Now some were there but they vanished (8) I have some left and my uh diamonds. (9) I have a whole, what do you call it? Thing of them, plus two big ones . . . (10) I got tired of them moving (11) So I was listening to the uh TV (12) And said, "they're mine." (13) So I got those. (14) I uh happened to be uh kind of a bind. (15) There's not much I could say. (16) I know who it is, you know (17) And I don't want the rest of them lost. (18) It was somebody I live near. (19) My husband worked with a lady at the bank. (20) Uh, I didn't know what to think for a while 21. And things started being real good (22) And then all of a sudden that horrible thing out in the uh, where they killed all those people and children. (23) Well, I covered that (24) And they were mad (25) So they took everything away from me they could.

Topic Maintenance: Variable. Most of the utterances (1–21) relate to stamps or diamonds and the topics of a thief and related statements. In utterances 22 to 24 there is a digression from the main topic. There may have been some associations for the speaker between the two sets of events, but these associations are not evident to or even inferable by the listener. In the final utterance the speaker returns to the general topic of theft.

Event Sequencing: Impaired. Few events are presented; a plausible sequence cannot even be reconstructed.

Informativeness: Inappropriate. Not enough information is present for the listener to make sense of the narrative. The listener cannot determine whether the narrative is elaborated because it is so incoherent. There is more evaluation (utterances 1, 3, 10, 14, 15, 16, 17, 20, 21, 22, 24, 25) than description (utterances 7, 8, 9, 18, 19) and action (utterances 5, 6, 7b, 11, 12, 13, 22, 23, 25).

Referencing: Variable. The speaker is able to provide definite referents, such as "stamps" (utterance 2), "diamonds" (utterance 8), "husband" (utterance 19) and "bank" (utterance 19). However, it is not clear how these referents fit into the narrative. She uses indefinite noun references that reduce discourse coherence (utterances 7, 8, 9, 21, and 22). Indefinite pronouns (utterances 5, 6, 7, 12, 13, 22, 24, and 25) and omitted or misrepresented references (utterances 17 and 23) are also evident.

Conjunctive Cohesion: Appropriate. The speaker uses a variety of conjunctions for semantic purposes: coordination (utterances 12, 17, etc.), temporal sequencing (utterance 6), disjuncture (utterance 7), causality (utterances 13 and 25), and for pragmatic functions: beginning of discourse (utterance 2) and change of focus (utterance 11).

Fluency: Appropriate. The narrative is fluent.

Intervention Goals. Intervention is difficult because we do not know whether the speaker has the potential to improve her narrative discourse abilities given her cognitive disabilities. Initial steps might focus on discourse in brief structured tasks, such as scripts and procedural discourse. The speaker could briefly describe a routine activity. Later more unstructured discourse tasks might be incorporated into an intervention program.

> *Example from a 31-year-old European North American man with traumatic brain injury (from our files)*
> **Interviewer:** Have you ever gotten lost?
>
> **Client:** (1)[*Long pause*] About the only really good time I can remember getting lost was in West Virginia. (2) Me and my brother had been walking into the woods one day, (3) And we found a pig in the woods. (4) A pig. (5) Pig got out of my uncle's . . . pig, uh . . . (6) So we found a pig around. (7) And then we found out that we did get lost. (8) So we went walking through the woods for about two hours, until it got really dark. (9) Then we found a house and went back home. (10) But during the time that we were lost, we were really scared 'cause we didn't think we were going to make it back. (11) And I got all upset and started crying like a little wimp. (12) And I didn't think we were goin' make it back. (13) But we did. (14) It was a little traumatic for me . . . (15) 'Cause I didn't think we were going to make it.

Topic Maintenance: Appropriate. All the sentences relate to one specific experience.

Event Sequencing: Appropriate. Events are told in a plausible, chronological order.

Informativeness: Variable. While we have most of the information we need to make basic sense of the story, the speaker is unable to retrieve the word *pen* or *stock* in utterance 5. In terms of elaboration, the speaker is impaired. We wish to know what happened when they found the pig. Did he make noise or run away? What happened to the pig after the speaker and his brother finally got back home? Did the speaker and his brother live near the uncle or were they visiting? What house did they find?

In terms of narrative ingredients, the speaker is also variable. He includes some description (utterance 8), but not much. We do not know anything about the size or appearance of the pig, for example. There is action (utterances 3, 5, 6, 9) and lots of evaluation (utterances 1, 8, 10, 11, 12, 14).

Referencing: Variable. The speaker specifies that he was with his brother (utterance 2). (Although he uses ungrammatical, colloquial English construction to do so, this does not represent impairment.) Thereafter, he grammatically uses the pronoun *we*. Similarly, the speaker introduces *a house* grammatically in utterance 9. However, there is a missing *the* article in reference to the pig (utterance 5), and use of *around* is unusual (utterance 6).

Conjunctive Cohesion: Appropriate. The speaker uses a number and variety of conjunctions for both semantic and pragmatic purposes. Specifically, he uses *and* for coordination (utterances 3, 11, 12), *and then* and *then* for temporal conjunction (utterances 7, 9), *So* and *'cause* for causal conjunction (utterances 8, 10, 15), and *But* for disjuncture—all appropriate semantic connections. He also uses *So* (utterance 6) and *But* (utterance 10) pragmatically to note his departures from chronology in a fashion that suggests he is aware of his impairments and is monitoring them.

Fluency: Variable. While the production is not entirely dysfluent, the speaker does struggle with this dimension (long pause at outset and in utterances 5 and 14). Utterance 5 is abandoned due to word-finding difficulties, but also contains redundant, nonevaluative reference to the pig.

Intervention Goals.   The goal for this speaker is to increase executive functioning. The narrator needs to be aware that his discourse is incomplete and requires elaboration. He needs to monitor his production and be aware of the discourse needs of the listener. Contingent queries will be useful.

> *Example from Mexican American man with traumatic brain injury (from our files)*
> **Interviewer:** Have you ever been in a car accident?
> **A:**   Yes, uhhuh. (1) We got off some tubes and, and . . . I don't know.
> **Interviewer:**   Yes, and what happened?

A: (2) I don't know. (3) Me—here she left me. . . .

Interviewer: They left you here?

A: Uhhuh.

Interviewer: Yes, Okay. Tell me more.

A: (4) And she left.

Interviewer: She left?

A: Uhhuh.

Interviewer: And what happened then?

A: (5) Well, I don't know. I haven't known.

Interviewer: You haven't known?

A: No.

Interviewer: No? Okay, good.

A: (6) That is what happened (7) and I haven't known about her since it has happened.

Interviewer: You don't know what happened?

A: No.

Interviewer: Okay, very good.

A: Yes . . . (8) because she left me here last night (9) and here is that she left me (10) and she herself left me.

Interviewer: Okay, good.

A: (11) And that is that she happened no more.

Interviewer: Okay.

Topic Maintenance: Appropriate. All utterances are related to one topic, the car accident.

Event Sequencing: Needs further study. No sequence is presented; events could not be ordered.

Informativeness: Inappropriate. This narrative does not have enough specific information, let alone elaboration. There is no description and the only type of evaluation is the use of negation.

Referencing: Inappropriate. We do not know who "she" is, and she is the most important participant beside the narrator.

Conjunctive Cohesion: Appropriate. The narrator uses *and, since,* and *because,* though this hardly helps him communicate, and the vagueness of the utterances connected make it impossible to determine the nature of the relationship encoded.

Fluency: Variable. While spoken false starts, internal corrections, and repetitions are at a minimum, the narrator seems unable to develop his thoughts.

Intervention Goals.   Informativeness and referencing are the most important goals for this speaker.

> ***Example from 19-year-old African American man with traumatic brain injury (from our files)***
>
> **Interviewer:**   Have you ever had anything stolen?
>
> **Client:**   My money was stolen. Fifty dollars.
>
> **Interviewer:**   Fifty dollars . . . Uh-huh.
>
> **Client:**   Yah, I was in the back of the truck with my cousin and he said he has it. So I went looking and looking and looking. I didn't find it. I beat him up.

Topic Maintenance: Appropriate. All utterances relate to the theft.

Event Sequencing: Appropriate. Several events are sequenced chronologically.

Informativeness: Inappropriate. Especially in view of African American culture's value for lengthy narration (see Chapter 4), this narrative lacks specific information, not to mention engaging elaboration. The narrator includes a bare minimum of actions ("looking"), description ("fifty dollars"), and evaluation ("I didn't find it"), but so scant as to come up deficient in this area, provided this narrative represents the upper limits of his ability.

Referencing: Appropriate so far as this slim passage is concerned.

Conjunctive Cohesion: Appropriate, minimally. One *and* and one *so* used appropriately.

Fluency: Appropriate.

Intervention Goals.   The speaker needs to increase the informativeness of his narration. Specific information, elaboration, description, and evaluation are all necessary.

11

Assessment and Intervention with Acquired Adult Discourse Impairments

Assessment Applications

Elicitation

The genre of personal narratives has been used successfully with adults who exhibit a variety of symptoms and disorders (Biddle, McCabe, & Bliss, 1996; Bliss, McCabe, & Miranda, 1998). This genre reflects a natural form of discourse that will lay the foundation for intervention (McCabe, 1995). Most adults with acquired communicative impairments are able to produce personal narratives. The exceptions are individuals with moderate and severe Broca's (nonfluent) aphasia who cannot link more than two utterances in an utterance and some patients with dementia who cannot produce a coherent message.

Prompts for personal narratives need to be relevant for adults. Some examples are presented in Chapter 1.

Analyses of Adult Narration

Narrative Profiles. Profiles are useful in assessing the narrative discourse abilities of adults. They can both be used to identify an adult's relative strengths and weaknesses and determine appropriate goals for intervention. The narrative assessment profile enables clinicians to identify and compare specific communicative abilities. Profiles have been completed for three narratives that have been produced by patients in the preceding chapters with Broca's aphasia (nonfluent) Wernicke's aphasia (fluent), and unspecified dementia (see the charts on pages 168–170).

A comparison of the three profiles reveals interesting similarities and differences among the speakers. The Broca's (nonfluent) and the Wernicke's (fluent) patients exhibited strengths in topic maintenance, event sequencing, and conjunctions. Informativeness and referencing were variable. Although the dimensions were impaired, different symptomatologies were evident for each speaker within the dimensions. Fluency was disrupted for adults with both types of aphasia, fluent and nonfluent aphasia. The types of dysfluency differ by the type of aphasia; that is, the patient with Broca's aphasia produced internal corrections, while the patient with Wernicke's aphasia produced false starts and many repetitions in a flowing manner (hence the term "fluent aphasia"). The adult with unspecified dementia exhibited strengths in conjunctive cohesion and fluency while the other dimensions were impaired to varying degrees.

Interrelatedness of Dimensions.   The NAP dimensions do not represent discrete independent aspects of discourse. They frequently overlap and influence each other, as well as nondiscourse-level aspects of language. For example, word finding deficits decrease referencing and fluency. Omitted references decrease informativeness. This interrelatedness of the dimensions will assist clinicians in identifying intervention goals. That is, focusing on one dimension may facilitate another narrative dimension. For example, informativeness and fluency may be improved when referencing is increased.

Discourse Genres.   A variety of discourse genres needs to be assessed in order to identify a speaker's communicative strengths. Conversation, scripts, and procedural discourse should be a part of assessment. The goal will be to determine the most suitable genre to begin intervention. While scripts and procedural discourse are not often functional, they may be a means to producing more complex forms of discourse. The NAP protocol can be used with all genres of discourse (see Chapter 7 for similar usage with children's genres).

Discourse Styles Used in the Home and Community.   An adult's preferred discourse style should be identified in assessment. For example, an African American speaker who enjoys using a performative style (see Chapter 4) or a Japanese speaker who values conciseness should be evaluated with respect to these cultural communicative values. In other words, these styles should not be considered to represent impairments for these speakers. Similar decisions need to be made for speakers from other cultures. In previous chapters, we described cultural communicative tendencies for speakers from diverse cultures. Assessment decisions should be made that respect the communicative values of speakers. Clinicians need to find out from family members information about a speaker's communicative styles before the onset of the disorder.

Use of Interpreters.   The use of interpreters in assessment is somewhat controversial. While they have knowledge of a speaker's first language, they are not trained to assess language behavior. They may be used in situations in which professionals do not have sufficient knowledge of an individual's first language. If used, interpreters should be trained to carefully provide the clinician with the exact utterances that a speaker has produced. It is a common tendency for some adults to fill in missing words or correct the grammar of a speaker.

Intervention Applications

The goals for intervention are determined partially by an adult's potential to improve narrative coherence. Narrative discourse may not be an appropriate goal for some patients. For example, individuals with moderate to severe Broca's aphasia will most likely be unable to produce the extensive connected discourse that is required for narration. Some individuals with dementia may not have the ability to construct, organize, and monitor a narrative. Patients with progressive neurological and mental disorders also may not be able to respond to narrative intervention.

Critical to the success of an intervention program is the support of family members and caregivers in adult facilities. Professionals need to consult with individuals who live and work with a patient so that they can model, encourage, and shape narrative attempts. Intervention cannot be successful in a clinical vacuum.

Intervention that is designed to enhance narrative discourse may need to begin with facilitating less challenging forms of discourse. Improvement of conversational discourse may be an initial step for some adults (in particular those exhibiting signs of Broca's aphasia). The dimensions of NAP (with the possible exception of event sequencing, depending on the topic of conversation) can be used to assess the coherence of conversation. Individuals who cannot maintain a topic (e.g., those with severe Wernicke's aphasia or dementia) may need to learn this dimension in conversation and scripts before they attempt narratives. They can master discourse coherence in scripts and procedural discourse before they attempt narratives. The former genres are less demanding than the latter one.

Intervention will also need to focus on receptive abilities for some patients. Some disruptions in topic maintenance may be the result of impaired comprehension or self-monitoring. Receptive skills are not the focus of this book but should be considered in a comprehensive treatment plan.

Intervention with narration should reflect the discourse styles prevalent in the home and community. With children, we advocated eliciting genres that are expected in schools in order to assist children academically. This recommendation is not relevant for adults. Trying to elicit narratives in a form different from the client's cultural norm seems useless, even alienating in therapy. For example, for some Spanish-speaking adults, family vignettes should be facilitated because this form of narration may be used in their home. For some Japanese speakers, brief narratives should be accepted, following the cultural values of the community. Clinicians will need to identify the most appropriate narrative style for each client, usually by consultation with family members.

Narrative Intervention Strategies

The intervention strategy of DIME (developed by the second author) is appropriate for most adults with communicative impairments. This procedure is reviewed below:

1. **D = Discourse Elicitation**
   The speaker attempts a narrative. If it is inappropriate, the clinician carries out the following steps:
2. **I = Identification**
   The professional asks directed questions in order to identify the aspects of the narrative that were not appropriate. The questions function to redirect the adult to the original topic. They may also serve to introduce referents that have not been previously identified and provide additional information that was missing. For example, if an adult omits a referent, the professional can ask the speaker to identify the referent by a pronoun or a proper name. If the adult does not maintain a topic, the clinician can ask questions as a means of redirecting the client to the original topic. If critical information is missing, the clinician can pose questions that identify what was omitted.
3. **M = Model**
   The clinician models the complete narrative or segments of the narrative as a means of focusing on the aspects that were originally produced inappropriately. For example, the clinician could begin by modeling setting or orientation information that was not originally included (e.g., "You had the car accident on Sunday evening in New Jersey"). The clinician could model appropriate referencing ("Your wife and nephew were in the car. They were not hurt").
4. **E = Elicited Production**
   The speaker is asked to produce segments of the original narrative. Narratives may be co-constructed, with the clinician and the speaker each relating parts of the narrative. Elicited production may also consist of the complete narratives or narratives that describe new topics. The amount of clinician support can gradually be decreased.

Intervention for Specific NAP Dimensions

Some of the intervention activities that are described in this section focus on discourse forms other than narrative, such as conversation or scripts. Their role is a prenarrative function—a bridge to narration. For some clients, easier forms of discourse need to be elicited before more challenging forms are attempted.

Topic Maintenance.   Some topics that are relevant to adults are banking, cooking, raising children, insurance, injuries, thefts, unusual animal experiences, and buying a house or car. One primary target of intervention should be monitoring of discourse. An individual needs to recognize when utterances diverge from the main topic. The professional can use verbal redirection techniques that direct the client to the original topic within discourse. The following exchange represents verbal redirection for topic maintenance:

> **Professional:** Tell me about why you came to the hospital.
>
> **Client:** I was brought in two days ago. My son just got engaged.
>
> **Professional:** You came to the hospital because you had a stroke. Why did you come to the hospital?

Some specific activities to foster topic maintenance are:

1. Have the client respond to simple and complex questions regarding a topic (e.g., "What does X have to do with what you were talking about?"). Although this task is not a monologic narrative one, it will enable a client to respond appropriately in conversation, an easier form of discourse than narrative.
2. Scripts and procedural discourse may be easier for some clients to master topic maintenance skills than narratives. Attempt these genres initially.

Event Sequencing.   In working with clients from cultures that value this dimension, professionals should highlight chronological sequencing of events. The following intervention strategies are relevant:

1. An effective means for enabling clients to sequence events is to use anchor points, such as *first, then, next,* and *last.* These words help to organize a speaker's thoughts.
2. An event can be segmented into separate units and then resequenced into a complete narrative. Model short passages with appropriate sequencing. Then have the client attempt to produce the narrative.
3. Have clients master scripts and procedural discourse before they attempt narratives.

Informativeness.   Speakers should be made aware when they do not provide enough information. They need to be informed of the consequences of omitting critical information. For example, omitting one's residence location when making a 911 call may delay professional response. Omission of descriptions, actions, and evaluations may cause a listener to become confused. Some therapeutic activities include:

1. Directed questions enable a speaker to add missing information and will increase informativeness. Simple questions are *who, what* and *when;* complex forms are *why* and *how.*
2. Clients can make phone calls that require that specific information be conveyed. Although this task does not necessarily produce a full, monologic narrative, it does serve to demonstrate the importance of including sufficient

information for the listener. Some examples: calling a repair shop to describe a faulty appliance or giving directions to one's house.

Referencing.   With middle-class clients from cultures that value explicit referencing, clinicians may want to work on introducing participants, events, and objects within a specific context.

1. Contexts need to be developed in which a referent is introduced and then is referenced. Have the client describe an event that includes one or more individuals. The client will need to refer back to the character in a specific context.
2. Have clients retell the plots of movies or books that have multiple characters. While this task is not common in daily discourse, it does enable them to focus on the need for appropriate referencing.

Conjunctive Cohesion.   This dimension should not receive focus early in intervention. Most adult patients are able to conjoin their utterances, as has been seen in the narratives in this book. A possible exception is patients with nonfluent or Broca's aphasia.

Fluency.   Dysfluencies are frequently associated with word retrieval deficits and are common in adult discourse impairments.

1. Activities for word finding are appropriate for many patients. Word retrieval strategies for adults are provided in other resources (e.g., Helms-Estabrooks, & Holland, 1998; Rosenbek, LaPointe, & Wertz, 1989).
2. Different genres on an identical topic (e.g., personal narratives, scripts, and procedural discourse) should be used to achieve flexible word retrieval. An individual can describe one banking experience (personal narrative), specific procedures to deposit money (e.g., procedural discourse), and routine banking procedures (e.g., script).

Examples of Narrative Intervention

In this section we will describe narrative intervention (see charts on pages 168–170) with respect to the three speakers whose narratives were presented in Chapter 10. These procedures should be applicable for other adults with similar impairments.

The goals for the patient with Broca's aphasia (p. 151) are to increase elaboration, especially description, and to elicit appropriate referencing.

Intervention should begin with scripts and easy forms of procedural discourse. The purpose of starting at this level is to use a less challenging form of discourse than narration. The clinician would encourage the speaker to describe procedures such as how to buy groceries or fill a car with gasoline. The DIME procedures would be used to model elaboration, description, and specific lexical use (these genres do not lend themselves to the use of evaluations and proper names). The aim is to enable the client to increase the informativeness of his or her messages.

After this level, the clinician would elicit short structured narratives. For example, "Tell me about one time you went to the movies" could be used as a prompt. The narrative should be segmented into small units and then reconstructed into a larger passage. Conjunctions could be highlighted to link the episodes. Later, the clinician could elicit more elaborate narratives that include a variety of people, multiple experiences, and different perspectives.

The goals for the first client with Wernicke's aphasia (p. 152, who talked about her stolen car) are to increase word retrieval and evaluation. Intervention procedures would follow traditional word retrieval procedures (Helms-Estabrooks & Holland, 1998; Rosenbek et al., 1989). Thematically based discourse should be implemented; the speaker would be encouraged to describe personal experiences in order to use effective word finding strategies. This speaker also needs to include evaluation in her discourse. She should be asked to describe people, objects, and internal states. Questions such as "How do you feel? and What did it look like?" could be posed.

Individuals such as the woman on page 156 with moderate to severe unspecified dementia have devastating discourse impairments. Narrative discourse might not be a suitable goal for intervention because it requires planning, organization, and monitoring that patients with this type of disorder may be incapable of carrying out. However, individuals with mild dementia may be able to narrate short passages, and this would be a desirable goal for their ongoing relationships with family and friends. Conversational discourse would be a first step for some patients because it is the most functional and useful. A speaker needs to be able to answer questions with responses that are on topic and coherent. Intervention could proceed from answering simple questions (e.g., *what, who, where*) to those that are more complex (e.g., *how, why*). If coherence is achieved at this level, scripts and procedural discourse can be elicited. Directed questions and verbal redirection may facilitate discourse coherence.

For the speaker with dementia in Chapter 10, the "stealing" experience should be segmented into separate units and then recombined into a larger event. The clinician should ask specific questions that would identify the major events of the experience. Questions such as "What was stolen? Where were they taken? Do you know who stole them? Did anything happen to the thief?" could be asked. The answers to these and other questions could be developed into a coherent narrative. The speaker should then try to relay this event to a new listener in shorter and then longer segments.

In summary, the narrative discourse impairments exhibited by the adults in this book and registered by NAP are varied and specific. Assessment should be structured to identify individuals' discourse profiles of strengths and weaknesses. Intervention should focus more on the general areas of discourse (e.g., topic maintenance, event sequencing, and informativeness) than on specific features (e.g., referencing). The speaker's premorbid communicative style must not be penalized and should be preserved in intervention. Family members and caregivers are critical to both assessment and intervention.

NARRATIVE ASSESSMENT PROTOCOL

Name of Client: _____ Diagnosis: <u>Broca's aphasia</u>

Cultural/Linguistic Background: <u>European North American man (p. 149)</u>

Narrative Aspect	Appropriate, Variable, Inappropriate, Needs Further Study	Description of Narrative Discourse
Topic Maintenance	Appropriate	All utterances are focused on one topic.
Event Sequencing	Appropriate	Events are properly sequenced.
Informativeness	Variable	Lacks elaboration and description but has action.
Referencing	Variable	Indefinite noun references are omitted or misrepresented ("blob"); some unspecified pronouns.
Conjunctive Cohesion	Appropriate	Only two conjunctions used.
Fluency	Variable	Two internal corrections.

Conclusions and recommendations: <u>The patient's narration is impaired. Intervention should be directed at increasing elaboration, description, and referencing.</u>

NARRATIVE ASSESSMENT PROTOCOL

Name of Client: _____ Diagnosis: <u>**Wernicke's aphasia**</u>

Cultural/Linguistic Background of Client: <u>**African American woman (p. 152)**</u>

Narrative Aspect	Appropriate, Variable, Inappropriate, Needs Further Study	Description of Narrative Discourse
Topic Maintenance	Appropriate	All utterances concern one topic.
Event Sequencing	Appropriate	Events in order.
Informativeness	Variable	No evaluation.
Referencing	Variable	Adequate pronoun and noun referencing; semantic and verbal paraphasias ("caught my head").
Conjunctive Cohesion	Appropriate	Both semantic and pragmatic purposes denoted.
Fluency	Inappropriate	False starts, repetitions.

Conclusions and recommendations: <u>The patient's narration abilities are impaired. Intervention should focus on increasing lexical referencing and the use of evaluation.</u>

NARRATIVE ASSESSMENT PROTOCOL

Name of Client: _____ Diagnosis: <u>Unspecified dementia</u>

Cultural/Linguistic Background: <u>European North American woman (p. 156)</u>

Narrative Aspect	Appropriate, Variable, Inappropriate, Needs Further Study	Description of Narrative Discourse
Topic Maintenance	Variable	One unrelated segment inserted into the narrative.
Event Sequencing	Inappropriate	Events not presented chronologically.
Informativeness	Inappropriate	Narrative is not coherent, though evaluation, description, and action are used.
Referencing	Variable	Some definite referents are used; use of indefinite noun and pronoun referents; some omitted or misrepresented references.
Conjunctive Cohesion	Appropriate	Use of a variety of connectives for semantic and pragmatic purposes.
Fluency	Appropriate	Absence of dysfluencies.

Conclusions and recommendations: <u>The patient's narrative abilities are severely impaired.</u>
<u>Intervention should initially focus on increasing discourse coherence in conversation, scripts,</u>
<u>and procedural discourse before narration is attempted.</u>

Part 4

Summary of NAP for Children and Adults

In this book, we have attempted to summarize extensive information on cultural differences in storytelling, age-related developments, and various individual disabilities, both congenital and acquired. Although we have subdivided the book in such a way that people seeking information on children can attend to the first eight chapters, while people seeking information on adults can attend to Chapters 1, 2, 9, 10, and 11, we do not want exaggerate the extent to which the book should be so subdivided. This last part, for example, should be read by everyone who is seeking to diagnose difficulty and who is mindful of and sensitive to cultural differences in narration. We also encourage clinicians working with adults from diverse cultures to read the chapters in the children's section that provide relevant information on their clients' cultural backgrounds.

We have covered a great deal of information and appreciate that accurately diagnosing narrative difficulty without misunderstanding cultural differences is a complex task. What follows are some summary charts that we hope will make the task more manageable. Please use these charts in conjunction with reading relevant chapters on culture (Chapters 3–6), as the charts are not intended to stand alone. The charts are:

1. Blank form for qualitative Narrative Assessment Profile used throughout this book
2. Summary Chart: NAP Dimensions for Four Ethnic Groups
3. Blank form for *quantitative* Narrative Assessment Profile, with informativeness weighted more than the other dimensions due to its importance, complexity, and vulnerability to deficit

4. Examples of scorings by ethnic group and dimension: What does appropriate, variable, and inappropriate use of various dimensions look like?

We conclude with our wish that this book helps us truly understand individuals from all cultures better than we have in the past.

NARRATIVE ASSESSMENT PROTOCOL

Name of Client: _____ Date of Birth: _____

Narrative Eliciter: _____ Cultural/Linguistic Background: _____

Narrative Aspect	Appropriate, Variable, Inappropriate, Needs Further Study	Description of Narrative Discourse
Topic Maintenance		
Event Sequencing		
Informativeness		
Referencing		
Conjunctive Cohesion		
Fluency		

Conclusions and recommendations: _____

_____

SUMMARY CHART: NAP DIMENSIONS FOR FOUR ETHNIC GROUPS

	European North American	*African American*	*Spanish-speaking American*	*Asian American*
Topic Maintenance	Single experience	Single experience or multiple, thematically related experiences	Single or multiple experiences; conversation-focused narration	Multiple (2–3) similar experiences in one narrative
Event Sequencing	Yes	Yes	Optional, de-emphasized	Optional, de-emphasized
Informativeness				
Police officer (specific experience)	Yes	Yes	Yes	Yes
Teacher (elaboration)	Provide details about single experience	Embellish facts, sometimes at great length	Focus on maintaining conversational flow	Combine several (2–3) similar experiences
Chef (description, action, evaluation)	All three	All three	All three, but actions de-emphasized	All three
Referencing	Explicit style preferred, except by some low SES groups, who prefer implicit style	Explicit style preferred, except by some low SES groups, who prefer implicit style	Pronouns sometimes omitted	Implicit style greatly preferred by all SES groups; omission of pronouns common, polite
Conjunction Cohesion	Yes	Yes	Yes	Yes
Fluency	Yes	Yes	Yes, but some ESL dysfluencies expected	Yes, but some ESL dysfluencies expected

NARRATIVE ASSESSMENT PROTOCOL: QUANTITATIVE VERSION

Name of Client: _____ Date of Birth: _____

Narrative Eliciter: _____ Cultural/Linguistic Background: _____

Narrative Aspect	Appropriate, Variable, Inappropriate, Needs Further Study	Description of Narrative Discourse
*Topic Maintenance	2 = All utterances on topic, culturally defined (A) 1 = Most on topic; off-topic associations, likes, dislikes, etc. (V) 0 = Most utterances are off-topic and/or topic is difficult to discern (I)	
*Event Sequencing	2 = All events in chronological order or acknowledged as out of order by conjunctions, etc., if culture values this (A) 1 = Most events chronologically ordered (V) 0 = No chronological ordering (I)	
*Informativeness: Police officer	2 = All specific information necessary to understand experience is provided or implied; credit should be given for easily inferred information (A) 1 = Most specific information provided but omissions of a few important points (V) 0 = Not enough information (I)	
*Informativeness: Teacher	2 = Culturally apt elaboration (A) 1 = Moderate elaboration (V) 0 = Only 1–2 statements at best (I)	

(continues)

NARRATIVE ASSESSMENT PROTOCOL: QUANTITATIVE VERSION (CONT.)

Name of Client: _____ Date of Birth: _____

Narrative Eliciter: _____ Cultural/Linguistic Background: _____

Narrative Aspect	Appropriate, Variable, Inappropriate, Needs Further Study	Description of Narrative Discourse
Informativeness: Chef	2 = All three ingredients (A) 1 = One missing ingredient (V) 0 = Two missing (I)	
*Referencing	2 = All references appropriate for culture and SES (A) 1 = Most pronouns used appropriately (V) 0 = Severely impaired referencing (I)	
Conjunctive Cohesion	2 = Variety used (A) 1 = Only *ands,* and *thens* (V) 0 = No conjunctions (I)	
Fluency	2 = Fluent (in both languages) 1 = A few dysfluencies 0 = Almost every utterance is dysfluent	
TOTAL (of 16 possible points)		

*Cultural variation in this dimension has been documented. See appropriate chapter and/or preceding summary chart for further explanation. Give full credit for cultural variation.

Conclusions and recommendations: _____

_____

Examples of Scorings by Ethnic Group and Dimension

	European North American			African American			Spanish-speaking American		
	A	**V**	**I**	**A**	**V**	**I**	**A**	**V**	**I**
Topic Maintenance	43 (TBI)	48 (ADHD)	41 (SLI)	63 (SLI)			82 (SLI)		
Event Sequencing	46 (HI)	43 (TBI)	41 (SLI)	63 (SLI)			82 (SLI)		
Informativeness	43 (TBI)	48 (ADHD)	41 (SLI)	55–60 (TL)	152 (WA)	63 (SLI)	73–77 (TL)	83 (SLI)	82 (SLI)
Referencing	36 (TL)	41 (SLI)	49 (Aut)	63 (SLI)	65 (HI)	66 (MR)	82 (SLI)	83 (SLI)	158 (TBI)
Conjunctive Cohesion	47 (MR)	41 (SLI)	49 (Aut)	63 (SLI)		66 (MR)	83 (SLI)		82 (SLI)
Fluency	47 (MR)	48 (ADHD)	43 (TBI)	63 (SLI)	154 (WA)	152 (WA)	82 (SLI)	158 (TBI)	86 (TBI)

Numbers = Pages where narrative examples can be found.   A = Appropriate; V = Variable; I = Inappropriate.

Diagnosis in parentheses:

   ADHD = Attention Deficit Disorder with Hyperactivity

      Aut = Autism

       HI = Hearing impairment

      MR = Mental retardation

      SLI = Specific Language Impairment

      TBI = Traumatic Brain Injury

       TL = Typical language

      WA = Wernicke's aphasia

Appendix

Parents as Teachers of Preliteracy Skills: An Intervention Study

Carole Peterson

Memorial University of Newfoundland
Psychology Department, St. John's, NF A1B 3X9
Tel: 709-737-7682; e-mail: carole@play.psych.mun.ca

Allyssa McCabe

University of Massachusetts at Lowell
Psychology Department, One University Ave., Lowell, MA 01854
Tel: 978-934-3968; e-mail: mccabeak@aol.com

Beulah Jesso

Memorial University of Newfoundland
Psychology Department, St. John's, NF A1B 3X9

Background

Parents are crucial members of every child's education team, the group of people who are responsible for educating the child from infancy to adulthood and preparing him or her with the skills necessary for future success. Lots of skills are involved, of course, from social-emotional maturity to academic skills. This section focuses on language and literacy skills.

Literacy is an important component of children's education; children with poor literacy skills have difficulties in school and are more likely to drop out at an early age. Numerous people have emphasized the important contribution parents make to their children's development of literacy by reading to them on a regular basis. However, many parents do not engage in such activity, perhaps because there are few if any books in the house, or because they themselves have poor literacy skills. Nevertheless, these parents can still play a vital role in helping their children learn the skills that underlie literacy, and teachers and other professionals can help them to do so.

Our recent intervention program showed how parents could help preschool-aged children learn some of the important preliteracy skills that have been shown to lay the foundation for later acquisition of literacy in school (Peterson, McCabe, & Jesso, 1999). This intervention program can be facilitated by professionals who work with the families of children, including teachers as part of their collaboration with parents.

The intervention program was based upon findings by researchers that a common everyday activity, namely talking about events that occurred sometime in the past, helps children learn the skills needed to create language about things that are not "here-and-now." These stories about real-life events help children learn how to organize their thoughts and to communicate about the "there-and-then." They help children knit together multiple sentences about a single topic, and they help them learn what kinds of information should be included in descriptions of these distant events. And all of these skills help lay a foundation upon which literacy is built (Dickinson, 1991; Reese, 1995; Snow, 1983). In fact, the storytelling or narrative skills of children before entering school have been found to be one of the best predictors of later school outcomes for those children who are at risk for academic and language problems (Paul & Smith, 1993).

The intervention program was also founded upon the research showing that the ways in which parents routinely talk with their children play a crucial role in children's development of narrative skills (Haden, 1998; McCabe & Peterson, 1991; Peterson & McCabe, 1992, 1994; Reese, Haden, & Fivush, 1993). Some parents extend each narrative topic being discussed, providing elaboration and lots of questions that elicit details about events and context. Other parents make little reference to the past event being discussed and ask only a few simple and redundant questions, switching from topic to topic quickly. These differences in parental style have been shown to influence both the quantity and quality of narratives produced by children.

Can we help parents talk to their children more effectively? Specifically, can we encourage parents to foster the sorts of storytelling skills that are helpful in school? Our intervention program's success provides a resounding "yes."

Components of Intervention

What are the ways in which parents can help children acquire these important preliteracy skills? The intervention program stresses the following key points:

1. **Talk to your child frequently and consistently about past experiences.**
2. **Spend a lot of time talking about each topic.**

3. Ask plenty of *who, what, when, where,* and *why* questions and few *yes/no* questions. As part of this, ask questions about the context or setting of the events, especially where and when they took place.
4. Listen carefully to what your child is saying and encourage elaboration.
5. Encourage your child to say more than one sentence at a time by using supportive responses (e.g., Uh-huh? Really? Yeah? You did?) or simply repeating what your child has just said.
6. Follow your child's lead. That is, talk about what your child wants to talk about, even if you would prefer not to.

The Intervention Program Itself

In this section we will describe the intervention program, focusing on what we did at each step. We recruited families of children in child-care centers when the children were between 3 and 4 years of age. All families in our program were supported by social assistance (Canadian welfare), and all lived in subsidized housing. Many were single-parent households.

The researcher who conducted the intervention program was a member of the culture to which the parents belonged, and so she knew what good stories were like in that culture. She was excellent at establishing rapport with the parents, and in fact on almost every visit she and the mother "had a cuppa" (cup of tea) in the kitchen.

The intervention program included the following steps. (Remember that this was a demonstration program, and so it included research components that allowed us to assess the effectiveness of the program. Specifically, there was a lot of pretesting and posttesting of both children's skills and parent behavior to see how they changed as a consequence of the program. Such evaluation components aren't crucial in other programs, but they allowed us to see whether this program was effective.) A summary of our intervention program is found in Table A.1.

First, the researcher visited the families at home. During this visit (which lasted 45 minutes to an hour), she established rapport with the families. She brought supplies for coloring, and she and the children colored while talking, as well as played in other ways. She also "had a cuppa" with the mother. Then she gave the mother a battery-powered tape recorder and asked her to talk to her child for half an hour about anything the pair wanted to talk about. She went back and collected the tape recorder a day or two later.

On a second visit a week later, after reestablishing rapport, she conducted a language assessment of the children by giving them the *Peabody Picture Vocabulary Test* (PPVT). She also talked with the children (while coloring), during which she asked the children about events that had happened in their lives. She gave them a number of standardized prompts, such as "One time I stepped on a bee and got stung. Have you ever gotten stung by a bee?" "Once I went to a birthday party at McDonald's. Have you ever been to a birthday party at McDonald's?" Such elicitation techniques have been found to be successful at encouraging narratives

TABLE A.1   *A Successful Research Intervention*

Session	Length	Content of Session
Initial home visit	45–60 minutes	Established rapport with children and parents.
		Left tape recorder for mother-child conversation.
2nd visit, 1 week later	1½ hour	PPVT assessment of child.
		Experimenter elicited narratives from child.
		Introduced mother to intervention program.
3rd visit, 1 week later	1½ hour	Gave mother a copy of our list of points.
		Played tapes, showed examples, role-played.
4th visit, 1 week later	45 minutes	Provided more feedback about prior role playing.
		Did more role playing.
Every 2 weeks for 1 year	10 minutes each	Telephone calls to provide encouragement to parents and reminders of our intervention points.

about past experiences in children (Peterson & McCabe, 1983). Once the children began narrating about a topic, the experimenter encouraged continuation by means of providing supportive responses such as "Uh-huh," "Yeah?" "Really?" and "and then what happened?" or repeating what the children had just said. As a consequence of the researcher's pretesting, we knew what the children's vocabulary and storytelling skills were like before the intervention started.

After the child assessment (which lasted 45 minutes to an hour), the researcher had tea with the mother, during which time she explained what researchers know about how children learn to tell stories, and in particular that parents' ways of talking to their children affect the quality and quantity of their storytelling. Parents who talk to their children a lot about the events in their children's lives and who ask them lots of questions that use specific question words *who, what, where, when,* and *why* have children who have better language skills and who learn to tell better stories. This is important because children with good storytelling or narrative skills have been found to do better in school. They are better able to express themselves, and, when they go to kindergarten, they are better able to reiterate what they have done when talking to the teacher. In short, these skills help children fit in better at school socially and academically. The researcher then talked with the mother about our list of six important points and asked if she would like to try to do these things over the next year. This discussion with the mother lasted approximately half an hour. We found mothers to be enthusiastic since they all wanted to help their children in any way they could.

A week later the researcher returned, and over tea she refreshed the mother's memory of our list of six points by giving her a copy of the list and talking about it. She also played tapes and passed out written transcripts of them. Some tapes were of mothers talking effectively to their children, while others were of mothers talking to their children in less effective ways. Such parents habitually had short conversations in which they frequently changed the topic of conversation. They often asked yes/no questions that did not encourage children to elaborate or even to talk at all. Then the mother and researcher engaged in role playing, which was tape-recorded. The researcher first played the part of the parent while the mother played the part of the child, and then they reversed roles. Then they listened to the tape of the role playing and talked about what they had done. An additional important component of this visit was talking to the mother about ways in which she could increase the amount of time she talked to her child about the events that occurred. The researcher helped the mother figure out times of the day when such narrative interaction could easily be incorporated, such as bath time, bedtime, mealtime, or when traveling in a car or bus. This visit lasted about 1½ hours.

Prior to the next visit, the researcher listened to the tapes and developed more feedback to give the mother. The next visit with the mother took place about a week later, during which time they reviewed the previous visit and listened again to the role-playing session that they had done. Then they did more role playing (playing both parts and taping again) and discussed their new tape so that the researcher could provide more feedback. This visit lasted about 45 minutes.

During the next year, the researcher called the participating mothers every two weeks and asked them how the program was going. She asked them what they were doing and how they were talking to their child. What sorts of things had they been talking about? What points from our list did they remember to use? If the researcher noticed that they forgot to mention one of our points, she reminded them of it. Lots of positive feedback was given to the mothers about what they were doing. This telephone conversation lasted about 10 to 15 minutes. Every two months, the researcher revisited the mothers and discussed what they were doing, and she left a tape recorder to get another sample of the mothers talking with their children. Thus, over the course of the year the mothers received regular reminders of the six key points of the intervention program as well as lots of opportunities for positive feedback.

Overall, this intervention program involved approximately four hours of working with each mother to teach her ways of talking with her child that were effective in helping their language and storytelling skills, plus 45 to 60 minutes of assessment of the initial skills of the child. This was followed by regular but short telephone calls and visits to provide the mothers with reminders and feedback. In short, little time is required per parent (see Table A.1). And yet, this minimal investment of time had large payoffs in terms of the children's skills.

Effect of the Intervention Program

To effectively assess the impact of the intervention program, we had a control group of mothers who were recruited the same way as the intervention mothers were. In fact, we initially developed our group of participating mothers and then randomly assigned them to either the intervention or control group. The control group mothers were visited on a regular basis as well, and their children had the same assessments of their language and storytelling skills as did the children of the intervention group mothers. However, the control mothers were told that we were interested in how mothers and children talked together and how the children's language skills change with age. At the end of the year of intervention, both intervention and control group mothers were given tape recorders and asked to talk to their children. As well, the PPVT was administered a second time and a different researcher (who did not know which group each child belonged to) talked with the children and elicited stories from them so that we could assess their skills. There was no contact with the parents for a year, and then we had yet another researcher talk with all of the children again to elicit more stories from them, so that we could measure the children's storytelling skills a full year after the intervention program ended.

How well did the intervention program do? First, children whose mothers had participated in the intervention program substantially increased their scores on the PPVT by the end of the intervention, relative to what they had been during the pretest. In contrast, the control group children had PPVT scores almost identical to their previous ones. Since children's PPVT scores are one of the best indicators of children's overall language skills, this suggests that the intervention program substantially helped the children's language development.

A year later, we could see the impact of our program on children's narrative skill. The children in the intervention group were telling lots more narratives and these narratives were longer. In addition, their narratives contained much more information and they were providing the sorts of "there-and-then" context setting (i.e., when and where events took place) that seem to be particularly important for later literacy acquisition. Although these improvements in story telling skills were not apparent at the end of the intervention, they were present a year later.

This delay is probably because it takes time for such fundamental language skills to change, and it also takes time for parents to acquire the habits of regularly talking to their children in the optimal ways that we fostered rather than in the ways that they had used prior to the intervention program. Over the year of intervention we found that the intervention mothers indeed did substantially change their ways of talking to their children, whereas the control group mothers showed no change at all. And with time, these changes in ways of talking with their children by the intervention mothers led to substantial improvements in their children's language skills. (A detailed description of our scoring categories as well as the data from both groups are found in Peterson, McCabe, & Jesso, 1999).

Research into Practice

This intervention program is cost-effective in that it does not take very much time per parent. Yet it helps parents develop ways of talking with their children that are helpful in fostering language skills and in particular the sorts of skills that seem to lay the foundation for later literacy acquisition. Furthermore, working with parents rather than directly with the children undoubtedly helps other children in the same families, since these same patterns of parent-child talk are likely to be applied to future children as well as the target children. Although in the past we have interacted directly with the children themselves in the ways that we have fostered with parents, we have found it to be much more effective to work with parents, since there are so many times of the day when parents can incorporate one-to-one talk with their children about events in the children's lives.

In Table A.2, we outline a potential intervention program that can be implemented with small groups of parents. During the first group meeting, the facilitator establishes rapport and then introduces the program and explains the importance of the storytelling skills that the program emphasizes. The facilitator gives the parents a handout that lists the six points of our intervention program. Tapes of both effective and less effective parent-child conversations are played and discussed. Typed transcripts of these tapes are handed out to the parents. (A copy of the tapes and transcripts we used can be obtained from us.) The parents then enact the roles of both parents and children, using the points we emphasize. These role-playing performances are discussed among the group. At the end of the session, parents are asked to record themselves talking with their children. Most families probably have a tape recorder, but if none is available, the facilitator should loan one to the family. This first session would last approximately two hours.

TABLE A.2   *Research into Practice*

Session	Length	Content of Session
1st group meeting	2 hours	Establish rapport with parents.
		Introduce program and explain importance.
		Play tapes, show examples, and have parents role-play.
		Ask parents to record themselves talking with children at home.
2nd group meeting	2 hours	Listen to parent tapes and provide feedback.
		More role playing with feedback.
Every other week	10 minutes each	Telephone calls to provide encouragement to parents and reminders of our intervention points.

At the second group meeting, everyone listens to the parent tapes and gives feedback. This is followed by more role playing and feedback. Subsequently, the facilitator telephones the parents every other week for a year in order to remind them about the points of the program and support their efforts (see Table A.2).

Conclusions

Children need to acquire considerable skill in many aspects of language before they can be expected to learn how to read and write. Much research demonstrates that parental involvement is essential for children's language acquisition. Research also demonstrates how parents can become involved in helpful ways. One of the most important ways that parents can be encouraged to help their children's language acquisition is to encourage them to talk at length about experiences they have had. Our research demonstrates that such an intervention with parents significantly improved their children's ability to tell a narrative, as well as expanded their vocabulary—two very strong predictors of reading achievement in later years. Even parents without optimal literacy skills themselves can be encouraged to do this sort of activity on a regular basis. Teachers might consider this a new kind of homework for children. Finally, the parents we worked with found the intervention to be fun as well as helpful. Children's personal narratives are a rich source of information about the child's feelings, about how they understand what things have happened to them, and of the various roles they play (hero, victim, jokester, etc.), and parents readily respond to these delights. What surprises teachers and parents alike is that such talk is not just talk—it is an excellent, essential preparation for reading and writing.

References

Dickinson, D.K. (1991). Teacher agenda and setting: Constraints on conversation in preschools. In A. McCabe & C. Peterson (Eds.), *Developing narrative structure* (pp. 255–301). Hillsdale NJ: Erlbaum.

Haden, C.A. (1998). Reminiscing with different children: Relating maternal stylistic consistency and sibling similarity in talk about the past. *Developmental Psychology, 34,* 99–114.

McCabe, A., & Peterson, C. (1991). Getting the story: A longitudinal study of parental styles in eliciting oral personal narratives and developing narrative skill. In A. McCabe & C. Peterson (Eds.), *Developing narrative structure* (pp. 217–253). Hillsdale, NJ: Erlbaum.

Paul, R., & Smith, R.L. (1993). Narrative skills in 4-year-olds with typical, impaired, and late developing language. *Journal of Speech and Hearing Research, 36,* 592–598.

Peterson, C., & McCabe, A. (1983). *Developmental psycholinguistics: Three ways of looking at a child's narrative.* New York: Plenum.

Peterson, C., & McCabe, A. (1992). Parental styles of narrative elicitation: Effect on children's narrative structure and content. *First Language, 12,* 299–321.

Peterson, C., & McCabe, A. (1994). A social interactionist account of developing decontextualized narrative skill. *Developmental Psychology, 30,* 937–948.

Peterson, C., McCabe, A., & Jesso, B. (1999). Encouraging narratives in preschoolers: An intervention study. *Journal of Child Language, 26,* 49–67.

Reese, E. (1995). Predicting children's literacy from mother-child conversations. *Cognitive Development, 10,* 381–405.

Reese, E., Haden, C.A., & Fivush, R. (1993). Mother-child conversations about the past: Relationships of style and memory over time. *Cognitive Development, 8,* 403–430.

Snow, C.E. (1983). Literacy and language: Relationships during the preschool years. *Harvard Educational Review, 53,* 165–189.

References

Abouzeid, M.P., & McClurg, J. (under review), "We ought to be talking to each other": High school students map out a narrative strategy.

Adler, S. (1979). *Poverty children and their language: Implications for teaching and treating*. New York: Grune & Stratton.

Ancona, G. (1993). *Pablo remembers: The fiesta of the Day of the Dead*. New York: Lothrop, Lee and Shepard.

Atkin, S.B., (1993). *Voices from the fields: Children of migrant farmworkers tell their stories*. Boston: Little, Brown.

Azuma, H. (1986). Why study child development in Japan? In H. Stevenson, H. Azuma, & K. Hakuta (Eds.), *Child development and education in Japan*. New York: Freeman.

Bamberg, M. (1987). *The acquisition of narratives*. Berlin: Mouton de Gruyter.

Barry, A.K. (1991). Narrative style and witness testimony. *Journal of Narrative and Life History, 1*(4), 281–294.

Bayles, K.A., Kasniak, A.W., & Tomoeda, C.K. (1987). *Communication and cognition in typical and aging and dementia*. San Diego: College-Hill.

Beals, D.E., & Snow, C.E. (1994). "Thunder is when the angels are upstairs bowling": Narratives and explanations at the dinner table. *Journal of Narrative and Life History, 4*(4), 331–352.

Bellinger, D.C., Wypij, D., Kuban, K.C.K., Rappaport, L.A., Hickey, P.R., Wernovsky, G., Jonas, R.A., & Newburger, J.W. (1999). Developmental and neurological status of children at 4 years of age after heart surgery with hypothermic circulatory arrest or low-flow cardiopulmonary bypass. *Circulation, 100*, 526–532.

Berman, R.A., & Slobin, D.I. (1994). *Relating events in narrative: A crosslinguistic developmental study*. Hillsdale, NJ: Erlbaum.

Biddle, K.R., McCabe, A., & Bliss, L.S. (1996). Narrative skills following traumatic brain injury in children and adults. *Journal of Communication Disorders, 29*(6), 447–469.

Bishop, D.V.M., & Edmundson, A. (1987). Language-impaired four year olds: Distinguishing transient from persistent impairment. *Journal of Speech and Hearing Disorders, 52*, 155–173.

Bliss, L.S. (1993). *Pragmatic language intervention*. Eau Claire, WI: Thinking Publications.

Bliss, L.S., Covington, Z., & McCabe, A. (1999). Assessing the narratives of African American children. *Current Issues in Communication Sciences and Disorders, 26*, 164–165.

Bliss, L.S., McCabe, A., & Mahecha, N. (2000). Bilingual narratives of Hispanic children with and without language impairments. Paper presented at the Annual Convention of the American Speech-Hearing-Language Association. Washington, DC.

Bliss, L.S., McCabe, A., & Miranda, A.E. (1998). Narrative assessment profile: Discourse analysis for school age children. *Journal of Communication Disorders, 31*, 347–363.

Bloom, L., Rocissano, L., & Hood, L. (1976). Adult-child discourse: Developmental interaction between information processing and linguistic interaction. *Cognitive Psychology, 8,* 521–552.

Bloom, R.L., Borod, J.C., Obler, L.K., & Gerstman, L.J. (1993). Suppression and facilitation of pragmatic performance: Effects of emotional content on discourse following right and left brain damage. *Journal of Speech and Hearing Research, 36,* 1227–1235.

Brice, A. (1994). Spanish or English for language impaired Hispanic children? In D.N. Ripich and N.A. Creaghead (Eds.), *School discourse problems* (2nd ed.; pp. 133–154). San Diego: Singular Publications.

Brinton, B., & Fujiki, M. (1984). Development of topic manipulation skills in discourse. *Journal of Speech and Hearing Research, 27,* 350–358.

Brown, R. (1973). *A first language: The early stages.* Cambridge, MA: Harvard University Press.

Bruner, J.S. (1983). *Children's talk: Learning to use language.* New York: Norton.

Bruner, J.S. (1986). *Actual minds, possible worlds.* Cambridge, MA: Harvard University Press.

Burt, B.S., & McCabe, A. (1996). Chameleon writers?: Narrative styles in written story books. In A. McCabe (Ed.), *Chameleon readers: Teaching children to appreciate all kinds of good stories.* New York: McGraw-Hill.

Campbell, L.R. (1996). Issues in service delivery to African American children. In A.G. Kiamhi, K.E. Pollock, J.L. Harris (Eds.), *Communication development and disorders in African American children* (pp. 73–94). Baltimore, MD: Paul H. Brookes.

Cardebat, D., Demonet, J., & Doyon, B. (1993). Narrative discourse in dementia. In H. Brownell & Y. Joanette (Eds.), *Narrative discourse in neurologically impaired and typical aging adults* (pp. 316–323). San Diego: Singular Publishing.

Cazden, C. (1985). Classroom discourse. In M.C. Wittrock (Ed.), *Research on teaching* (3rd ed.; pp. 432–463). New York: Macmillan.

Champion, T.B. (1995). *A description of narrative development and production among African American English child speakers.* Unpublished dissertation, University of Massachusetts, Amherst, MA.

Champion, T.B. (1998). "Tell me somethin' good": A description of narrative structures among African American children. *Linguistics and Education, 9,* 251–286.

Champion, T.B., Katz, L., Muldrow, R., & Dail, R. (1999). Storytelling and storymaking in an urban preschool classroom: Building bridges from home to school culture. *Topics in Language Disorders, 19*(3), 52–67.

Champion, T.B., Seymour, H., & Camarata, S. (1995). Narrative discourse of African American children. *Journal of Narrative and Life History, 5,* 333–352.

Chang, C.J. (1994). Chinese children's narrative structure. Unpublished paper presented at Harvard University, Cambridge, MA.

Chapman, S.B., Culhane, K.A., Levin, H.S., Harward, H., Mendelsohn, D., Ewing-Cobbs, L., Fletcher, J.M., & Bruse, D. (1992). Narrative discourse after closed head injury in children and adolescents. *Brain and Language, 43,* 42–65.

Charon, R. (1993). Medical interpretation: Implications of literary theory of narrative for clinical work. *Journal of Narrative and Life History, 3*(1), 79–98,

Chenery, H.J., & Murdoch, B.E. (1994). The production of narrative discourse in response to animations in persons with dementia of the Alzheimer's type: Preliminary findings. *Aphasiology, 8,* 159–171.

Chenery, L.R., & Canter, G.J. (1990). Informational content and cohesion in the discourse of Alzheimer's disease. Paper presented at the Annual Convention of the American Speech-Language and Hearing Association, Seattle, WA.

Cheng, L.L. (1993). Asian-American cultures. In D.E. Battle (Ed.), *Communication disorders in multicultural populations* (pp. 38–77). Boston: Andover-Medical Publishers.

Clancy, P.M. (1986). The acquisition of communicative style in Japanese. In B.B. Schieffelin & E. Ochs (Eds.), *Language socialization across cultures* (pp. 213–250). New York: Cambridge University Press.

Colby, D., & Erwin, K. (2001). Cultural variation: Cambodian and Caucasian children's narratives. Unpublished paper, Lowell, MA: University of Massachusetts Lowell.

Craddock-Willis, K., & McCabe, A. (1996). Improvising on a theme: Some African American traditions. In A. McCabe (Ed.), *Chameleon readers: Teaching children to appreciate all kinds of good stories* (pp. 98–115). New York: McGraw-Hill.

Crago, M.B. (1994). Ethnography and language socialization: A cross-cultural perspective. *Cross-cultural perspectives in language assessment and intervention.* Gaithersburg, MD: Aspen.

Crais, E.R., & Lorch, N. (1994). Oral narratives in school-age children. *Topics in Language Disorders, 14,* 13–28.

Culatta, B., Page, J., & Ellis, J., (1983). Story retelling as a communicative performance screening tool. *Learning, Speech, and Hearing in the Schools, 4,* 66–74

Cummins, J. (1984). *Bilingualism and special education: Issues in assessment and pedagogy.* Austin, TX: Pro-Ed.

Cummins, J. (1991). Interdependence of first- and second-language proficiency in bilingual children. In E. Bialystok (Ed.), *Language processing in bilingual children* (pp. 70–89). Cambridge: Cambridge University Press.

Damico, J.S. (1985). Clinical discourse analysis: A functional approach to language assessment. In C.S. Simon (Ed.), *Communication skills and classroom success* (pp. 165–206). San Diego, CA: College-Hill Press.

Damico, J.S., Oller, J.W., & Storey, M.E. (1983). The diagnosis of language disorders in bilingual children: Pragmatic and surface-oriented criteria. *Journal of Speech and Hearing Disorders, 48,* 385–394.

Damico, J.S., Smith, M.D. & Augustine, L.E. (1996). Multicultural populations and language disorders. In M.D. Smith & J.S. Damico (1996), *Childhood language disorders* (pp. 272–299). New York: Thieme Medical Publishers.

Dasinger, L., & Toupin, C. (1994). *Relating events in narrative: A crosslinguistic developmental study.* Hillsdale, NJ: Erlbaum.

Day, J.C. (1996). *Population projections of the United States by age, sex, race, and Hispanic origin: 1995 to 2050.* U.S. Bureau of the Census, Current Population Reports, P25-1130. U.S. Washington, DC: U.S. Government Printing Office.

Deese, J. (1984). *Thought into speech: The psychology of a language.* Englewood Cliffs, NJ: Prentice-Hall.

DeHirsch, K., Jansky, J.J., & Langford, W.J. (1966). *Predicting reading failure.* New York: Harper & Row.

Delpit, L.D. (1988). The silence of dialogue: Power and pedagogy in educating other people's children. *Harvard Educational Review, 58*(3), 280–298.

Dennis, M., & Barnes, M.A. (1990). Knowing the meaning, getting the point, bridging the gap, and carrying the message: Aspects of discourse following closed head injury in childhood and adolescence. *Brain and Language, 39,* 428–446.

DeSanti, S., Koengih, L., Obler, L.K., & Goldberger, J. (1994). Cohesive devices and conversational discourse in Alzheimer's disease. In R.L. Bloom, L.K Obler, S. DeSanti, & J.S. Erlich (Eds.), *Discourse analysis and application studies in adult clinical populations* (pp. 201–215). Hillsdale, NJ: Lawrence Erlbaum Associates.

Dickinson, D.K., & Tabors, P. (2001). *Beginning literacy with language*. Baltimore, MD: Brookes.

Doi, T. (1973). *The anatomy of dependence*. Trans. J. Bester. Tokyo: Dodansha International (Original title: *Amae nokozo*, published by Kobundo, 1971).

Dube, E.F. (1982). Literacy, cultural familiarity, and "intelligence" as determinants of story recall. In U. Neisser (Ed.), *Memory observed*. San Francisco, CA: Freeman.

Ellis, D.G. (1983). Language, coherence, and textuality. In R.T. Craig & K. Tracy (Eds.), *Conversational coherence: Form, structure and strategy* (pp. 222–240). Beverly Hills: Sage Publications.

Ervin-Tripp, S. (1979). Children's verbal turn-taking. In E. Ochs & B. Schieffelin (Eds.), *Developmental pragmatics*. New York: Academic Press.

Fazio, B.B., Naremore, R.C., & Connell, P.J. (1996). Tracking children from poverty at risk for specific language impairment: A 3-year longitudinal study. *Journal of Speech and Hearing Research, 39,* 611–624.

Feagans, L. (1982). The development and importance of narratives for school adaptation. In L. Feagans & D.C. Farran (Eds.), *The language of children reared in poverty* (pp. 95–116). New York: Academic Press.

Feagans, L., & Applebaum, M.I. (1986). Validation of language subtypes in learning disabled children. *Journal of Experimental Psychology, 78,* 358–364.

Flood, J., Lapp, D., & Flood, S. (1984). Types of writing found in the early levels of basal reading programs: Preprimers through second grade readers. *Annals of Dyslexia, 34,* 241–255.

Flood, J., Lapp, D., & Nagel, G. (1991). An analysis of literary works in district core reading lists. *National Reading Conference Yearbook, 40,* 269–275.

Folstein, M., Folstein, S., McHugh, P. (1975). Mini-mental state. A practical method for grading the cognitive state of patients for the clinician. *Journal of Psychiatric Research, 12,* 189–198.

Foster, M. (1995). Talking that talk: The language of control, curriculum, and critique. *Linguistics and Education, 7*(2), 129–150.

Foster, S. (1986). The development of discourse topic skills in infants and young children. *Topics in Language Disorders, 5*(2), 31–45.

Frederiksen, C.H., & Stemmer, B. (1993). Conceptual processing of discourse by a right hemisphere brain-damaged patient. In H. Brownell & Y. Joanette (Eds.), *Narrative discourse in neurologically impaired and typical aging adults* (pp. 239–278). San Diego: Singular Publishing.

Garcia, R. (1987). *My Aunt Otilia's spirits/Los espiritus de mi Tia Otilia*. San Francisco, CA: Children's Book Press.

Gardner, M.F. (1983). *Expressive one-word picture vocabulary test*. Novato, CA: Academic Therapy Publications.

Garza, C.L. (1990). *Family pictures: Cuadros de familia*. San Francisco, CA: Children's Book Press.

Gee, J.P. (1991a). Memory and myth: A perspective on narrative. In A. McCabe & C. Peterson (Eds.), *Developing narrative structure* (pp. 1–25). Hillsdale, NJ: Lawrence Erlbaum Associates.

Gee, J.P. (1991b). A linguistic approach to narrative. *Journal of Narrative and Life History, 1,* 15–39.

George, K.P., & Johnson, A.F. (1995). Selected discourse process in acute right hemisphere stroke. Poster presented at the annual convention of the American Speech-Language Hearing Association, Orlando, FL.

German, D.J. (1992). Word-finding intervention for children and adolescents. *Topics in Language Disorders, 13*(1), 33–50.

German, D., & Simon, S. (1991). Analysis of children's word-finding skills in discourse. *Journal of Speech and Hearing Research, 34,* 309–316.

Gleason, J.B., & Ratner, N.B. (1998). *Psycholinguistics* (2nd ed.). New York: Harcourt Brace.

Glosser, G. (1993). Discourse production patterns in neurologically impaired and aged populations. In H. Brownell & Y. Joanette (Eds.), *Narrative discourse in neurologically impaired and typical aging adults* (pp. 191–252). San Diego: Singular Publishing.

Glosser, G., & Deser, T. (1990). Patterns of discourse production among neurological patients with fluent language disorders. *Brain and Language, 40,* 67–88.

Glosser, G., Wiener, M., & Kaplan, E. (1988). Variations in aphasic language behaviors. *Journal of Speech and Hearing Disorders, 53,* 115–124.

Goldman, R., & Fristoe, M. (2000). *Goldman Fristoe Test of Articulation 2.* Circle Pines, MN: American Guidance Service.

Graesser, A., Golding, J.M., & Long, D.L. (1991). Narrative representation and comprehension. In R. Barr, M.L. Kamil, P.B. Mosenthal, & P.D. Pearson (Eds.), *The handbook of reading research* (Vol. 2; pp. 171–205). New York: Longman.

Grafman, J., Thompson, K., Weingartner, H., Martinez, R., Lawlor, B.A., & Sunderland, T. (1991). Script generation as an indicator of knowledge representation in patient's with Alzheimer's disease. *Brain and Language, 40,* 344–458.

Graybeal, C.M. (1981). Memory for stories in language-impaired children. *Applied Psycholinguistics, 2,* 269–283.

Griffith, P.L., Ripich, D.N., & Dastoli, S.L. (1986). Story structure, cohesion, and propositions in story recalls by learning disabled and non-disabled children. *Journal of Psycholinguistic Research, 15*(6), 539–549.

Grosjean, F. (1982). *Life with two languages.* Cambridge, MA: Harvard University Press.

Gutiérrez-Clellen, V.F. (1996). Language diversity: Implications for assessment. In K.N. Cole, P.S. Dale, & D.J. Thal (Eds.), *Assessment of communication and language* (pp. 29–56). Baltimore, MD: Paul H. Brookes.

Gutiérrez-Clellen, V.F. (1999). Language choice in intervention by bilingual children. *American Journal of Speech-Language Pathology, 8,* 291–302.

Gutiérrez-Clellen, V.F., & Heinrichs-Ramos, L. (1993). Referential cohesion in the narratives of Spanish-speaking children: A developmental study. *Journal of Speech and Hearing Research, 36,* 559–567.

Gutiérrez-Clellen, V.F., & Iglesias, A. (1992). Causal coherence in the oral narratives of Spanish-speaking children. *Journal of Speech and Hearing Research, 35,* 363–372.

Gutiérrez-Clellen, V.F., Restrepo, M.A., Bedore, L., & Peña, E. (2000). Language sample analysis in Spanish speaking children: Methodological considerations. *Language, Speech, and Hearing Services in Schools, 31,* 88–98.

Hadley, P.A. (1998). Language sampling protocols for eliciting text-level discourse. *Language, Speech, and Hearing Services in Schools, 29,* 132–147.

Halliday, M.A.K., & Hasan, R. (1976). *Cohesion in English.* New York: Longman.

Hansen, C.L. (1978). Story retelling used with average and learning disabled readers as a measure of reading comprehension. *Learning Disability Quarterly, 1,* 62–69.

Harris, R.J., Lee, D.J., Hensley, D.L., & Schoen, L.M. (1988). The effect of cultural script knowledge on memory for stories over time. *Discourse Processes, 11,* 413–431.

Hartley, L.L., & Jensen, P.J. (1991). Narrative and procedural discourse after closed head injury. *Brain Injury, 5,* 267–285.

Hartley, L.L., & Jensen, P.J. (1992). Three discourse profiles of closed-head injury speakers: Theoretical and clinical implications. *Brain Injury, 6,* 271–282.

Heath, S.B. (1982). What no bedtime story means: Narrative skills at home and at school. *Language in Society, 11,* 49–76.

Heath, S.B. (1983). *Ways with words: Language, life and work in communities and classrooms.* Cambridge, England: Cambridge University Press.

Heath, S.B. (1986). Taking a cross-cultural look at narratives. *Topics in Language Disorders, 7,* 84–94.

Hedberg, N.L., & Westby, C.E. (1993). *Analyzing storytelling skills. Theory to Practice.* Tucson, AZ: Communication Skill Builders.

Heller, R.B., Dobbs, A.R., & Rule, B.G. (1992). Communicative function in patients with questionable Alzheimer's disease. *Psychology and Aging, 7,* 395–400.

Helms-Estabrooks, N., & Holland, A. (1998). *Approaches to the treatment of aphasia.* San Diego: Singular Publishing Group.

Hemphill, L. (1989). Topic development, syntax, and social class. *Discourse Processes, 12,* 267–286.

Hemphill, L., Uccelli, P., Willenberg, I., & Bellinger, D. (2001, April). Do narrative delays persist in children with early corrective heart surgery? Poster presentation at the Society for Research in Child Development. Minneapolis, MN.

Hemphill, L., Uccelli, P., Winner, K., & Chang, C. (2002). Narrative discourse in young children with histories of early corrective heart surgery. *Journal of Speech, Language, and Hearing Research.*

Hester, E.J. (1996). Narratives of young African American children. In A.G. Kamhi, K.E. Pollock, & J.L. Harris (Eds.), *Communication development and disorders in African American children: Research, assessment, and intervention* (pp. 227–245). Baltimore, MD: Paul H. Brookes.

Hinds, J. (1984). Topic maintenance in Japanese narratives and Japanese conversational interaction. *Discourse Processes, 7,* 465–482.

Hirschler, J.A. (1994). Preschool children's help to second language learners. *The Journal of Educational Issues of Language Minority Students, 14,* 227–239.

Hood, L., & Bloom, L. (1979). What, when, and how about why: A longitudinal study of early expressions of causality. *Monographs of the Society for Research in Child Development, 44,* No. 6.

Hough, M.S. (1990). Narrative comprehension in adults with right and left hemisphere brain damage: Theme organization. *Brain and Language, 23,* 26–33.

Hudson, J.A., & Shapiro, L.R. (1991). From knowing to telling: The development of children's scripts, stories, and personal narratives. In A. McCabe & C. Peterson (Eds.), *Developing narrative structure* (pp. 89–136). Hillsdale, NJ: Erlbaum.

Hughes, D., McGillivray, L., & Schmidek, M. (1997). *Guide to narrative language: Procedures for assessment.* Eau Claire, WI: Thinking Publications.

Hurston, Z.N. (1935; 1990). *Mules and men.* New York: Harper & Row.

Hymes, D. (1981). *"In vain I tried to tell you": Studies in Native American ethnopoetics.* Philadelphia: University of Pennsylvania Press.

Hymes, D. (1982). Narrative form as a "grammar" of experience: Native Americans and a glimpse of English. *Journal of Education, 2,* 121–142.

Hyon, S., & Sulzby, E. (1992). Black kindergartners' spoken narratives: Style, structure and task. Paper presented at the annual meeting of the American Educational Research Association, San Francisco, CA.

Hyon, S., & Sulzby, E. (1994). African American kindergartener's spoken narratives: Topic associating and topic centered styles. *Linguistics and Education, 6,* 121–152.

Hyter, Y.D. (1994). *Across channel description of reference in the narratives of African American Vernacular English speakers.* Unpublished doctoral dissertation. Philadelphia: Temple University.

Hyter, Y.D., & Westby, C.E. (1996). Using oral narratives to assess communicative competence. In A.G. Kamhi, K.E. Pollock, & J.L. Harris (Eds.), *Communication development and disorders in African American children: Research, assessment, and intervention* (pp. 247–275). Baltimore, MD: Paul H. Brookes.

Invernizzi, M.S., & Abouzeid, M.P. (1995). One story map does not fit all: A cross-cultural analysis of children's written story retellings. *Journal of Narrative and Life History, 5*(1), 1–19.

Irwin, J.W. (1980). The effects of linguistic cohesion on prose comprehension. *Journal of Reading Behaviour, 12,* 325–332.

Ito, T. (1986). Speech dysfluencies and acquisition of syntax in children 2–6 years old. *Folia Phoniatica, 38,* 310–315.

John, V.P., & Berney, J.D. (1968). Analysis of story retelling as a measure of the effects of ethnic content in stories. In J. Helmuth (Ed.), *The disadvantaged child: Head Start and early intervention* (Vol. 2). New York: Brunner/Mazel.

Johnston, J.J. (1982). Narratives: A new look at communication problems in older language impaired children. *Language, Speech, and Hearing Services in Schools, 13,* 144–155.

Johnston, J.R. (1982). Narratives: A new look at communication problems in older language-disordered children. *Language, Speech, and Hearing Services in Schools, 13,* 144–155.

Jones, F. (1999). Personal narratives profiles of African American preschoolers. Unpublished student paper. University of Houston, Houston, TX.

Jordan, F.M., & Murdoch, B.E. (1990). Linguistic status following closed head injury in children: A follow-up study. *Brain Injury, 4,* 147–154.

Jordan, F.M., Murdoch, B.E., & Buttsworth, D.L. (1991). Closed-head-injured children's performance on narrative tasks. *Journal of Speech and Hearing Research, 34,* 572–582.

Kaderavek, J.N., & Sulzby, E. (2000). Narrative production by children with and without Specific Language Impairment: Oral narratives and emergent readings. *Journal of Speech, Language, and Hearing Research, 43,* 34–49.

Kayser, H. (1995). Bilingualism, myths, and language impairments. In H. Kayser (Ed.), *Bilingual speech-language pathology: An Hispanic focus* (pp. 185–206). San Diego: Singular Publishing Group.

Kayser, H. (1995a). Intervention with children from linguistically and culturally diverse backgrounds. In M. Fey, J. Windsor, & S. Warren (Eds.), *Language intervention preschool through the elementary years* (pp. 315–332). Baltimore, MD: Paul Brookes.

Kayser, H. (1995b). Assessment of speech and language impairments in bilingual children. In H. Kayser (Ed.), *Bilingual speech-language pathology: An Hispanic focus* (pp. 243–264). San Diego: Singular.

Kempler, D., Curtiss, S., & Jackson, C. (1987). Syntactic preservation in Alzheimer's disease. *Journal of Speech and Hearing Research, 30,* 343–350.

Kernan, K. (1977). Semantic and expressive elaboration in children's narratives. In S. Ervin-Tripp & C. Mitchell-Kernan (Eds.), *Child discourse* (pp. 91–119). New York: Academic Press.

Kintsch, W., & Greene, E. (1978). The role of culture-specific schemata in the comprehension and recall of stories. *Discourse Processes, 1,* 1–13.

Labov, W. (1972). *Language in the inner city: Studies in the Black English Vernacular.* Philadelphia: University of Pennsylvania Press.

Lawrence, V.W., & Shipley, E. (1996). Parental speech to middle- and working-class children from two racial groups in three settings. *Applied Psycholinguistics, 17,* 233–255.

Lebra, T.S. (1986). *Japanese patterns of behavior* (5th ed.). Honolulu: University of Hawaii Press.

Liles, B. (1985a). Cohesion in the narratives of normal and language-disordered children. *Journal of Speech and Hearing Research, 28,* 123–133.

Liles, B. (1985b). The production and comprehension of narrative discourse in normal and language disordered children. *Journal of Communication Disorders, 18,* 409–427.

Liles, B.Z. (1987). Episodic organization and cohesive conjunctions in narratives of children with and without language disorder. *Journal of Speech and Hearing Research, 30,* 185–186.

Liles, B.Z. (1993). Narrative discourse in children with language disorders and children with typical language: A critical review of the literature. *Journal of Speech and Hearing Research, 36,* 868–882.

Liles, B.Z., Coelho, C.A., Duffy, R.J., & Zalagens, M.R. (1989). Effects of elicitation procedures on the narratives of typical and closed head-injured adults. *Journal of Speech and Hearing Disorders, 54,* 356–366.

Liles, B.Z., Duffy, R.J., Merritt, D.D., & Purcell, S.L. (1995). Measurement of narrative discourse ability in children with language disorders. *Journal of Speech and Hearing Research, 38,* 415–425.

Long, S.H. (1994). Language and bilingual-bicultural children. In V.A. Reed (Ed.), *An introduction to children with language disorders* (2nd ed.; pp. 290–317). New York: Maxwell Macmillan.

Lucas, E.V. (1980). *Semantic and pragmatic language disorders.* Rockville, MD: Aspen.

MacLachlan, B., & Chapman, R. (1988). Communication breakdowns in normal and language learning-disabled children's conversation and narration. *Journal of Speech and Hearing Disorders, 53,* 2–7.

Maeno, Y. (2000). *Acquisition of Japanese oral narrative style by native English-speaking bilinguals.* Unpublished doctoral dissertation, Cambridge, MA: Harvard University.

Mainess, K.J., Champion, T.B., & McCabe, A. (2002, in press). Telling the unknown story: Complex and explicit narration by African American preadolescents—Preliminary examination of gender and socioeconomic issues. *Linguistics in Education.*

Manavathu, M., & Bliss, L.S. (1998, November). Personal narratives profiles of African American preschoolers. Poster presented at the annual convention of the American Speech, Hearing and Language Association. San Antonio, TX.

Marsh, N.V., & Knight, R.G. (1991). Behavioral assessment of social competence following severe head injury. *Journal of Clinical and Experimental Neuropsychology, 13,* 729–740.

McCabe, A. (1991). Editorial. *Journal of Narrative and Life History, 1*(1), 1–2.

McCabe, A. (1995). Evaluation of narrative discourse skills. In K.N. Cole, P.S. Dale, & D.J. Thal (Eds.), *Assessment of communication and language* (pp. 121–142). Baltimore: Paul Brookes.

McCabe, A. (1996). *Chameleon readers: Teaching children to appreciate all kinds of good stories.* New York: McGraw-Hill.

McCabe, A., & Peterson, C. (1985). A naturalistic study of the production of causal connectives by children. *Journal of Child Language, 14*(2), 375–382.

McCabe, A., & Peterson, C. (1991). Getting the story: A longitudinal study of parental styles in eliciting narratives and developing narrative skill. In A. McCabe and C. Peterson, (Eds.), *Developing narrative structure* (pp. 217–254). Hillsdale, NJ: Lawrence Erlbaum Associates.

McCabe, A., & Rollins, P.R. (1994). Assessment of preschool narrative skills: Prerequisite for literacy. *American Journal of Speech-Language Pathology: A Journal of Clinical Practice, 3*(1), 45–56.

McConaughy, S.H. (1985). Good and poor readers' comprehension of story structure across different input and output modalities. *Reading Research Quarterly, 20*(2), 219–232.

McDonald, S. (1992). Communication disorders following closed head injury: New approaches to assessment and rehabilitation. *Brain Injury, 6*, 283–292.

McGann, W., & Schwartz, A. (1988). Main character in children's narratives. *Linguistics, 26*, 215–233.

McGregor, K., & Leonard, L. (1989). Facilitating word finding skills of language-impaired children. *Journal of Speech and Hearing Disorders, 54*, 141–147.

McGregor, K.K. (2000). The development and enhancement of narrative skills in a preschool classroom: Towards a solution to clinician-client mismatch. *American Journal of Speech-Language Pathology, 9*, 55–71.

McKeogh, A.M. (1987). Stages in storytelling: A neo-Piagetian analysis. Paper presented to the Biennial Meeting of the Society for the Study of Behavioral Development, Tokyo.

Meltzi, G. (2000). Cultural variations in the construction of personal narratives: Central American and European American mothers' elicitation styles. *Discourse Processes, 30*(2), 153–177.

Melzi, G. (1997). *Developing narrative voice: Conversations between Latino mothers and their preschool children.* Unpublished doctoral dissertation. Boston: Boston University.

Menig-Peterson, C. (1975). The modification of communicative behavior in preschool-aged children as a function of the listener's perspective. *Child Development, 46*, 1015–1018.

Menig-Peterson, C., & McCabe, A. (1978). Children's orientation of a listener to the context of their narratives. *Developmental Psychology, 74*, 582–592.

Mentis, M.L., & Prutting, C.A. (1991). Analysis of topic as illustrated in a head-injured and typical adult. *Journal of Speech and Hearing Research, 34*, 583–595.

Mentis, M.L., Briggs, J., & Gramigna, G.G. (1995). Discourse topic management in senile dementia of the Alzheimer's type. *Journal of Speech and Hearing Research, 38*, 1054–1066.

Menyuk, P., Chesnick, J., Liebergott, J.W., Korngold, B., D'Agostino, R., & Belanger, A. (1991). Predicting reading problems in at-risk children. *Journal of Speech and Hearing Research, 34*, 893–903.

Merritt, D.D., & Liles, B.Z. (1987). Story grammar ability in children with and without language disorder: Story generation, story retelling, and story comprehension. *Journal of Speech and Hearing Research, 30*, 539–552.

Merritt, D.D., & Liles, B.Z. (1989). Narrative analysis: Clinical applications of story generation and story retelling. *Journal of Speech and Hearing Disorders, 54*, 429–438.

Michaels, S. (1981). Sharing time: Children's narrative styles and differential access to literacy. *Language and Society, 10*, 423–441.

Michaels, S. (1991). The dismantling of narrative. In A. McCabe & C. Peterson (Eds.), *Developing narrative structure* (pp. 303–352). Hillsdale, NJ: Lawrence Erlbaum Associates.

Michaels, S., & Foster, M. (1985). Peer to peer learning: evidence from a student run sharing time. In A. Jaggar & M.T. Smith-Burke (Eds.), *Observing the language learner* (pp. 143–158). Newark, DE: International Reading Association.

Miller, L. (1990). The roles of language and learning in the development of literacy. *Topics in Language Disorders, 10*, 423–442.

Miller, P.J., & Sperry, L.L. (1988). Early talk about the past: The origins of conversational stories of personal experience. *Journal of Child Language, 15*, 293–316.

Minami, M. (1990). Children's narrative structure: How do Japanese children talk about their own stories? Special qualifying paper. Harvard Graduate School of Education, Cambridge, MA.

Minami, M. (1996). Japanese preschool children's and adults' narrative discourse competence and narrative structure. *Journal of Narrative and Life History, 6*(4), 349–373.

Minami, M. (1996). Japanese preschool children's narrative development. *First Language, 16,* 339–363.

Minami, M. (2001, personal communication). Conjunctions in Japanese narration.

Minami, M., & McCabe, A. (1991). Haiku as a discourse regulation device: A stanza analysis of Japanese children's personal narratives. *Language in Society, 20,* 577–600.

Minami, M., & McCabe, A. (1995). Rice balls versus bear hunts: Japanese and European North American family narrative patterns. *Journal of Child Language, 22,* 423–446.

Minami, M., & McCabe, A. (1996). Compressed collections of experiences: Some Asian American traditions. In A. McCabe (Ed.), *Chameleon readers: Teaching children to appreciate all kinds of good stories* (pp. 72–97). New York: McGraw-Hill

Miranda, A.E. (1995). *Semantic and pragmatic analyses of narrative discourse in language impaired and nonimpaired children.* Unpublished doctoral dissertation. Cambridge, MA: Graduate School of Education of Harvard University.

Miranda, A.E., McCabe, A., & Bliss, L.S. (1994). Jumping around and leaving things out: Assessing impaired narration. Miniseminar presented at the annual convention of the American Speech-Language Hearing Association, New Orleans, LA.

Miranda, A.E., McCabe, A., & Bliss, L.S. (1998). *Assessment of narrative skills of school age children.* Unpublished manuscript.

Miranda, A.E., McCabe, A., & Bliss, L.S. (1998). Jumping around and leaving things out: A profile of the narrative abilities of children with specific language impairment. *Applied Psycholinguistics, 19*(4), 647–656.

Miranda, A.E., McCabe, A., & Bliss, L.S. (1998). Jumping around and leaving things out: Dependency analysis applied to the narratives of children with specific language impairment. *Applied Psycholinguistics, 19,* 657–668.

Mortensen, L. (1992). A transivity analysis of discourse in dementia of the Alzheimer's type. *Journal of Neurolinguistics, 7,* 309–321.

Moya, K.L., Benowitz, L.I., Levine, D.N., & Finkelstein, S. (1986). Covariant deficits in visuospatial abilities and recall of verbal narrative after right hemisphere stroke. *Cortex, 22,* 381–397.

Myers, P. (1993). Narrative expressive deficits associated with right-hemisphere damage. In Brownell, H.H. & Joanette, Y. (Eds.), *Narrative discourse in neurologically impaired and typical aging adults* (pp. 279–296). Singular Publishing Groups: San Diego.

Myers, P.S. (1994). Communication disorders associated with right-hemisphere brain damage. In R. Chapey (Ed.), *Language intervention strategies in adult aphasia* (3rd ed.; pp. 513–534). Baltimore: Williams & Wilkins.

Naremore, R.C., Densmore, A.E., & Harman, D.R. (1995). *Language intervention with school-aged children.* San Diego: Singular Publishing Group.

Nelson, N.W. (1999). *Childhood language disorders in context: Infancy through adolescence* (2nd ed.). Boston: Allyn and Bacon.

New Standards Project. (1999). *Reading and writing grade by grade: Primary literacy standards for kindergarten through third grade.* www.ncee.org

New Standards Project (2001). *Speaking and listening for preschool through third grade.* www.ncee.org

Nicholas, L.E., & Brookshire, R.H. (1993). A system for quantifying the informativeness and efficiency of the connected speech of adults with aphasia. *Journal of Speech and Hearing Research, 36,* 338–350.

Nicholas, L.E., & Brookshire, R.H. (1995). Presence, completeness, and accuracy of main concepts in the connected speech of non-brain-damaged adults and adults with aphasia. From a sample alone. *Journal of Speech and Hearing Research, 38,* 145–156.

Nicholas, M., Obler, L.K., Albert, M.L., & Helm-Estabrooks, N. (1985). Empty speech in Alzheimer's disease and fluent aphasia. *Journal of Speech and Hearing Research, 28,* 405–410.

Norris, J., & Hoffman, P. (1990). Language intervention within naturalistic environments. *Language, Speech & Hearing Services in the Schools, 21,* 72–84.

Norris, J., & Hoffman, P. (1993). *Whole language intervention for school-age children.* San Diego, CA: Singular Publishing Group.

O'Brien, T. (1990). *The things they carried.* New York: Penguin.

Obler, L.K., & Albert, M.L. (1981). Language in the senile patient and the elderly aphasic patient. In M. Sarno (Ed.), *Acquired aphasia* (pp. 385–398). New York: Academic Press.

Obler, L.K., & Albert, M.L. (1984). Language in aging. In M.L. Albert (Ed.), *Clinical neurology of aging* (pp. 245–253). New York: Oxford University Press.

Olley, L. (1989). Oral narrative of normal and language-impaired school-aged children. *Australian Journal of Human Communication Disorders, 17,* 43–65.

Ovadia, R., Hemphill, L., Winner, K., & Bellinger, D. (2000). Just pretend: Participation in symbolic talk by children with histories of early corrective heart surgery. *Applied Psycholinguistics, 21,* 321–340.

Owens, R.E. (1996). *Language development.* Boston: Allyn and Bacon.

Owens, R.E. (1999). *Language disorders: A functional approach to assessment and intervention* (3rd ed.). Boston: Allyn and Bacon.

Paek, M. (1988). *Aekyung's dream.* San Francisco, CA: Children's Book Press.

Paul, R. (2001). *Language disorders from infancy through adolescence.* St. Louis: Mosby.

Paul, R., & Smith, R.L. (1993). Narrative skills in 4-year-olds with typical, impaired, and late-developing language. *Journal of Speech and Hearing Research, 36,* 592–598.

Peréz, C. (1998). *The language of native Spanish and English speaking schizotypal college students.* Unpublished doctoral dissertation. Boston: University of Massachusetts Boston.

Perry, T., & Delpit, L. (1998). *The real ebonics debate.* Boston: Beacon.

Peterson, C., Jesso, B., & McCabe, A. (1999). Encouraging narratives in preschoolers: An intervention study. *Journal of Child Language, 26,* 49–67.

Peterson, C., Jesso, B., & McCabe, A. (1999). Encouraging narratives in preschoolers: An intervention study. *Journal of Child Language, 66*(2), 257–284.

Peterson, C., & McCabe, A. (1983). *Developmental psycholinguistics: Three ways of looking at a child's narrative.* New York: Plenum.

Peterson, C., & McCabe, A. (1987). The connective "and": Do older children use it less as they learn other connectives? *Journal of Child Language, 14*(2), 375–382.

Peterson, C., & McCabe, A. (1991). Linking children's connective use and narrative macrostructure. In A. McCabe & C. Peterson (Eds.), *Developing narrative structure* (pp. 29–53). Hillsdale, NJ: Lawrence Erlbaum Associates.

Peterson, C., & McCabe, A. (1991). On the threshold of the storyrealm: Semantic versus pragmatic use of connectives in narratives. *Merrill-Palmer Quarterly, 37*(3), 445–464.

Peterson, C., & McCabe, A. (1992). Parental styles of narrative elicitation: Effect on children's narrative structure and content. *First Language, 12,* 299–321.

Preece, A. (1987). The range of narrative forms conversationally produced by young children. *Journal of Child Language, 14,* 353–373.

Pritchard, R. (1990). The effects of cultural schemata on reading processing strategies. *Reading Research Quarterly, 25*(4), 273–295.

Propp, V. (1968). *Morphology of the folktale.* Austin, TX: University of Texas Press. (Originally published, 1928).

Prutting, C.A., & Kirchner, D. (1987). A clinical appraisal of the pragmatic aspects of language. *Journal of Speech and Hearing Disorders, 52*, 105–119.

Purcell, S., & Liles, B.Z. (1992). Cohesion repairs in the narratives of normal-language and language impaired school-aged children. *Journal of Speech and Hearing Research, 35*, 354–362

Purcell, S.L., & Liles, B.Z. (1992). Cohesion repairs in the narratives of normal-language and language-disordered school-age children. *Journal of Speech and Hearing Research, 35*, 354–362.

Reed, V. (1994). Assessment and diagnosis. In *An introduction to children with language disorders* (2nd ed.; pp. 415–441). New York: Merrill.

Ripich, D.N., & Griffith, P.L. (1988). Narrative abilities of children with learning disabilities and nondisabled children: Story structure, cohesion, and propositions. *Journal of Learning Disabilities, 2*(3), 165–173.

Ripich, D.N., & Terrel, B.Y. (1988). Patterns of discourse cohesion and coherence in Alzheimer's disease. *Journal of Speech and Hearing Disorders, 53*, 8–15.

Rodino, A., Gimbert, C., Peréz, C., Craddock-Willis, K., & McCabe, A. (1991, October). Getting your point across: Contrastive sequencing in low-income African American and Latino children's personal narratives. Paper presented at the 16th Annual Conference on Language Development, Boston University, Boston, MA.

Roman, M., Brownell, H.H., Potter, H.H., Siebold, M.S., & Gardner, H. (1987). Script knowledge in right hemisphere-damaged and in typical elderly adults. *Brain and Language, 31*, 151–170.

Rosen, H. (1985). *Stories and meaning.* Upper Montclair, NJ: Norton.

Rosenbek, J.C., LaPointe, L.L., & Wertz, R.T. (1989). *Aphasia: A clinical approach.* Boston: Little, Brown.

Roth, F.P. (1986). Oral narrative abilities of learning-disabled students. *Topics in Language Disorders, 7*, 21–30.

Roth, F.P., & Spekman, N.J. (1986). Narrative discourse: Spontaneously generated stories of learning-disabled and typically achieving students. *Journal of Speech and Hearing Disorder, 51*, 8–23.

Ruíz, N. (1989). An optimal learning environment for Rosemary. *Exceptional Children, 56*, 130–144.

Sabin, E.J., Clemmer, E.J., O'Connell, D.C., & Kaval, S. (1979). A pausological approach to speech development. In A.W. Siegman and S. Feldstein (Eds.), *Of speech and time: Temporal speech patterns in interpersonal context* (pp. 742–755). Hillsdale, NJ: Erlbaum.

Sakade, F. (Ed.). (1958). *Japanese children's favorite stories.* Rutland, VT: Charles E. Tuttle.

Schriffrin, D. (1987). *Discourse markers.* Cambridge, UK: Cambridge University Press.

Screen, R., & Anderson, N.B. (1994). *Multicultural perspectives in communication disorders.* San Diego, CA: Singular Publishing Group.

Sebastian, E., & Slobin, D.I. (1994). Development of linguistic forms: Spanish. In R.A. Berman & D.I. Slobin (Eds.), *Relating events in narrative: A crosslinguistic developmental study* (pp. 239–284). Hillsdale, NJ: Erlbaum.

Semel, E., Wiig, E., & Secord, W. (1995). *Clinical evaluation of language fundamentals-3.* San Antonio, TX: The Psychological Corporation.

Sherratt, S.M., & Penn, C. (1990). Discourse in a right hemisphere brain-damaged subject. *Aphasiology, 6*, 539–560.

Shigaki, I.S. (1987). Language and the transmission of values: implications from Japanese day care. In B. Fillion, C.N. Hedley, & E.C. DiMartino (Eds.), *Home and school: early language and reading.* Norwood, NJ: Ablex.

Silva, M.J., & McCabe, A. (1996). Vignettes of the continuous and family ties: Some Latino

American traditions. In A. McCabe (Ed.), *Chameleon readers: Teaching children to appreciate all kinds of good stories* (pp. 116–136). New York: McGraw-Hill.

Simmons-Mackie, N.N., & Damico, J.S. (1996). The contribution of discourse markers to the communicative competence in aphasia. *American Journal of Speech-Language Pathology, 5*, 37–43.

Ska, B., & Guenard, D. (1993). Narrative schema in dementia of the Alzheimer's type. In H. Brownell & Y. Joanete (Eds.), *Narrative discourse in neurologically impaired and typical aging adults.* San Diego: Singular Publishing.

Sleight, C., & Prinz, P.M. (1985). Use of abstracts, orientations, and codas in narration by language-disordered and nondisordered children. *Journal of Speech and Hearing Disorders, 50*, 361–371.

Smitherman, G. (1977). *Talkin' and testifyin': The language of Black America.* Boston: Houghton Mifflin.

Snow, C.E. (1983). Literacy and language: Relationships during the preschool years. *Harvard Educational Review, 53*, 165–189.

Snow, C.E., & Dickinson, D.K. (1990). Social sources of narrative skills at home and at school. *First Language, 10*, 87–103.

Stein, N., & Glenn, C. (1979). An analysis of story comprehension in elementary school children. In R. Freedle (Ed.), *New directions in discourse processing.* Hillsdale, NJ: Ablex.

Strong, C.J., & Shaver, J.P. (1991). Stability of cohesion in the spoken narratives of language-impaired and normally developing school-aged children. *Journal of Speech and Hearing Research, 34*, 95–111.

Stubbs, M. (1983). Discourse analysis: The sociololingistic analysis of natural language. Chicago: University of Chicago Press.

Tabors, P.O., & Snow, C.E. (2001). Young bilingual children and early literacy development. In S.B. Neuman & D.K. Dickinson (Eds.), *Handbook of early literacy research* (pp. 159–178).

Tabors, P.O., Snow, C.E., & Dickinson, D.K. (2001). Homes and schools together: Supporting language and early literacy development. In D.K. Dickinson & P.O. Tabors (Eds.), *Beginning literacy with language.* Baltimore, MD: Brookes.

Tomeoda, C.K., & Bayles, K.A. (1990). The efficacy of speech-language pathology intervention: Dementia. *Seminars in Speech and Language, 11*, 311–319.

Tomeoda, C.K., & Bayles, K.A. (1992). Longitudinal effects of Alzheimer disease on discourse production. *Alzheimer Disease and Associated Disorders, 7*, 223–236.

Tompkins, C.A. (1995). *Right hemisphere communication disorders: Theory and management.* Singular Press: San Diego.

Uccelli, P. (1997). *Beyond chronicity: Temporality and evaluation in Andean Spanish speaking children's narratives.* Unpublished qualifying paper. Cambridge, MA: Harvard Graduate School of Education.

Ulatowska, H.D., & Bond, S.A. (1983). Aphasia: Discourse considerations. *Topics in Language Disorders, 3*, 21–34.

Ulatowska, H.K., Allard, L., Donnell, A., Bristow, J., Haynes, S.M., Flower, A., & North, A.J. (1988). Discourse performance in subjects with demential of the Alzheimer's type. In H.A. Whitaker (Ed.), *Neuropsychological studies of non-focal brain damage: Trauma and dementia* (pp. 109–113). New York: Springer-Verlag.

Ulatowska, H.K., Allard, L., Donnell, A., Bristow, J., Haynes, S.M., Flower, A., & North. A.J. (1991). Discourse performance in subjects with dementia of the Alzheimer type. In H.A. Whitaker (Ed.), *Neuropsychological studies of non-focal brain damage: Trauma and dementia* (pp. 103–131). New York: Springer-Verlag.

Ulatowska, H.K., North, A.J., & Macaluso-Haynes, S. (1981). Production of narrative and procedural discourse in aphasia. *Brain and Language, 13*, 345–371.

U.S. Bureau of the Census. (1992). The Hispanic population in the United States: March, 1992. *Current Population Reports* (pp. 20–465). Washington, DC: U.S. Government Printing Office.

Van Djik, T. (1981). *Studies in the pragmatics of discourse.* The Hague: Mouton Publishers.

Vasquéz, O. (1989). *Connecting oral language strategies to literacy: An ethnographic study among four Mexican-American families.* Unpublished doctoral dissertation. Palo Alto, CA: Stanford University.

Wanska, S., & Bedrosian, J. (1985). Conversational structure and topic performance in mother-child interaction. *Journal of Speech and Hearing Research, 28,* 579–584.

Wapner, C.A., Hamby, S., & Gardner, H. (1981). The role of the right hemisphere in the apprehension of complex linguistic materials. *Brain and Language, 14,* 15–33.

Weaver, P.A., & Dickinson, D.K. (1982). Scratching below the surface structure: Exploring the usefulness of story grammars. *Discourse Processes, 5,* 225–243.

Westby, C.E. (1990). Ethnographic interviewing: Asking the right questions to the right people in the right ways. *Journal of Childhood Communication Disorders, 13,* 101–111.

Weylman, S.T., Brownell, H.H., Roman, M., & Gardner, H. (1989). Appreciation of indirect requests by left- and right brain-damaged patients: The effects of verbal context and conventionality of wording. *Brain and Language, 36,* 580–591.

Wong Fillmore, L. (1976). *The second time around: Cognitive and social strategies in second language acquisition.* Unpublished doctoral dissertation. Palo Alto: Stanford University.

Woodcock, R.W. (1981). *Woodcock Language Proficiency Battery: Spanish form.* Hingham, MA: Teaching Resources Corp.

Index